AF556766

Autologous Bone Plugs Fusion

To my wife Christine for her unending love, support and encouragement throughout the writing of this book.

Soo-Young Oh

Autologous Bone Plugs Fusion

Treatment for Lumbar Instability

- 3E Criteria
- Technical Operative Notes
- The Functioning of the Oh's Screw

107 figures, 4 tables, 2009

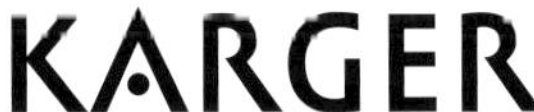

Basel · Freiburg · Paris · London · New York ·
Bangalore · Bangkok · Shanghai · Singapore · Tokyo · Sydney

Soo-Young Oh
Former Head of Neurosurgery Section
Department of Surgery
Kantonsspital Chur, Switzerland

Tutor, Department of Neurosurgery
University of Berne, Switzerland

Clinical Professor, Department of Neurosurgery
Korea University, Seoul, Korea

Former owner of St. Georg Clinic
Goldach, Switzerland

Address for correspondence:
Prof. Dr. med. Soo-Young Oh
Bondastr. 116
CH–7000 Chur (Switzerland)

Library of Congress Cataloging-in-Publication Data
Oh, Sooyoung.
Autologous bone plugs fusion : treatment for lumbar instability : 3E criteria, technical operative notes, the functioning of the Oh's screw / Soo-Young Oh.
p. ; cm.
The 3E triad complies with the Swiss health authorities quality standards -- Steps towards recognition -- Anatomical aspects of lumbar fusion -- Clinical consideration of instability -- Indication for operation -- Contraindication for plugs fusion -- History of Oh's temporary marking screw development -- Aspects of autologous bone plugs -- Operative technical procedure -- Routine postoperative checks (plug and screw) -- Expected effects -- Discussion -- History of transplantation surgery.
Includes bibliographical references and index.
ISBN 978–3–8055–9188–1 (hard cover : alk. paper)
1. Spine--Instability--Treatment. 2. Lumbar vertebrae. 3. Bone--Transplantation. 4. Autografts. I. Title.
[DNLM: 1. Lumbar Vertebrae--surgery. 2. Bone Screws. 3. Bone Transplantation. 4. Joint Instability--surgery. 5. Spinal Fusion. 6. Transplantation, Autologous. WE 750 O36a 2009]
RD771.I58O4 2009
617.4'71--dc22 2009023170

Disclaimer. The statements, opinions and data contained in this publication are solely those of the individual authors and contributors and not of the publisher and the editor(s). The appearance of advertisements in the book is not a warranty, endorsement, or approval of the products or services advertised or of their effectiveness, quality or safety. The publisher and the editor(s) disclaim responsibility for any injury to persons or property resulting from any ideas, methods, instructions or products referred to in the content or advertisements.

Drug Dosage. The authors and the publisher have exerted every effort to ensure that drug selection and dosage set forth in this text are in accord with current recommendations and practice at the time of publication. However, in view of ongoing research, changes in government regulations, and the constant flow of information relating to drug therapy and drug reactions, the reader is urged to check the package insert for each drug for any change in indications and dosage and for added warnings and precautions. This is particularly important when the recommended agent is a new and/or infrequently employed drug.

All rights reserved. No part of this publication may be translated into other languages, reproduced or utilized in any form or by any means electronic or mechanical, including photocopying, recording, microcopying, or by any information storage and retrieval system, without permission in writing from the publisher.

© Copyright 2009 by S. Karger AG, PO Box, CH–4009 Basel (Switzerland)
www.karger.com
Printed in Switzerland on acid-free and non-aging paper (ISO 9706) by Reinhardt Druck, Basel
ISBN 978–3–8055–9188–1
e-ISBN 978–3–8055–9189–8

Contents

Preface

An autologous transplantation fusion method with living tissue bone plugs has been performed optimally with no side reactions.

Minimally invasive operative procedures were performed for the treatment of lumbar column instability using substitution with original materials from the individual patient, as opposed to methods involving fixtures using materials formed from foreign substances.

Concerns of the triad 'E' criteria – economy, efficiency and expediency – are considered. Interdisciplinary collaboration provides great advantages for the patients and health care worldwide.

For patients who have allergic reactions to foreign substances, it is an ideal treatment as only autologous material is used.

The unilateral oblique posterior intervertebral body fusion (UOPIF) method, a technical fusion procedure, was developed by the author over the space of more than 15 years. In the meantime, this method, 'Oh's method', is being advised by insurance companies and particularly by actively lobbying patient members acknowledged by the Swiss Health Ministry and the insurance companies (health care must cover the costs).

The united ossified plug is a living, small and effective element which maintains its properties within the body indefinitely.

Introduction

A Long-Term Study

A new technical method using autologous bone plugs with unilateral oblique posterior interbody fusion (UOPIF) was researched and developed into a successful procedure. It is a minimally invasive alternative to spine instrumentation.

Patients were treated individually across a period of 18 years, from 1990 to 2008. 197 patients received autologous bone plugs at fusion for lumbar instability.

Spinal fixation with instrumentation is nowadays common practice and is a popular option for the treatment of segmental instability of the lumbar vertebral column.

Even though foreign body fixation has improved success rates in many disciplines, problems arise which include back pain caused by the instrumentation itself and allergic reactions and infection arising from the implantation of foreign bodies. Also, there is the issue of the high financial costs of the spine fixation instrumentation procedure.

However, there are now demonstrably significant advantages in utilizing the osseous consolidation artificial 'block spine' approach without foreign substances but with a living plug from the patient's own body.

The 3E Triad Complies with the Swiss Health Authorities Quality Standards

The Swiss Social Health Care Department and the Swiss Medical Association demand fulfillment of an essential 3E trial for optimal patient care for optimal treatment and coordination (fig. 1):

- Efficiency (patient)
- Expediency (surgeon)
- Economy (insurance and health care).

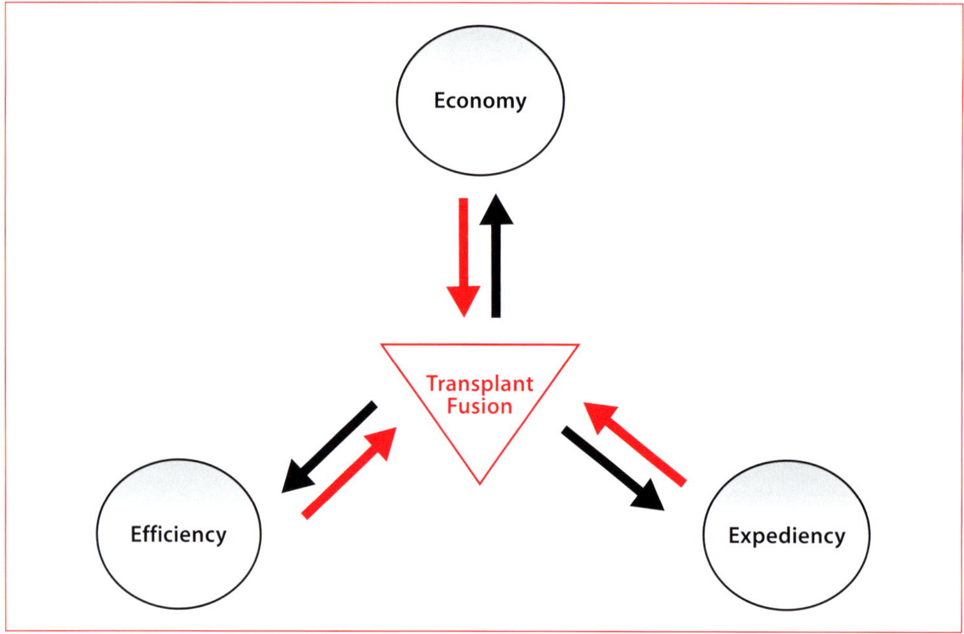

Fig. 1. The triad-E criteria expediency. Coordination of expediency-efficiency-economy has resulted in one of the best optimal medical care systems and is regarded as the standard in worldwide health care. The figure shows an example of autologous transplant treatment.

Two types of surgical care are given for lumbar instability:

(1) Foreign material – fixation-implantation-surgery.

(2) Organs or body part transplantation surgery.

Oh's method utilizing lumbar spondylodesis with autologous plugs has been already acknowledged by Swiss ELK, because of its compliance with the 3E Triad (see letter ELK; fig. 13).

During the last 20 years, surgeons have operated with various kinds of foreign body fixation using many different applications, materials and methods (fig. 2–5).

On the other hand, the only method used for fusion transplantations is:

- Autologous (skin, bone, etc.).

This treatment using the autologous approach is especially effective and has significant advantages.

Efficiency

For Patients

Before starting an operation, the surgeon thoroughly checks which method of treatment is to be followed for each individual patient, and informs and discusses the technique, alternative operations, secondary effects (fig. 3–5), and complications with the patients.

Comment

(Through Fusion Stabilization)

Well healed with living plug (fig. 2)

Lumbar segment stronger through stabilization

No foreign bodies

No foreign body reactions (see fig. 13)

Artificial block-vertebra-column has the appearance of a congenital anomaly (fig. 2).

The quality of the autologous bone plug transplantation bears no comparison to surgery with 'foreign' body implantation surgery.

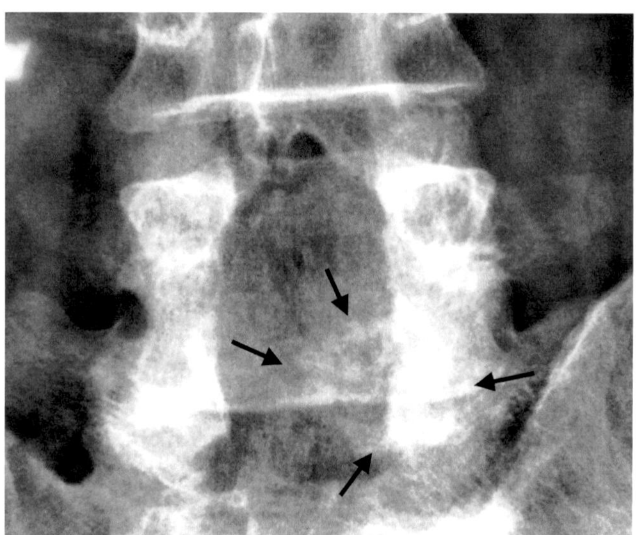

Fig. 2. Perfect and compact osseous consolidation with bone plug and vertebra body.

The author regards the choice of autologous material from the patient's own body as having the most satisfactory results in surgery compared to foreign body implantation.

In the course of his career, the author has seen many examples of less than successful procedures carried out by surgeons involving instrumentation with patients suffering from painful complications postoperatively (see published article, fig. 9).

There are considerable advantages for patients who are suffering. Among the therapeutic aspects of the use of their own body material are the prospects of hardly any complications and a good healing process (especially in patients with metal allergy).

Expediency

For Surgeons

Surgeons choose what kind of operation is to be done and which is best for the patient.

What kind of operation should be chosen – fixation or fusion?

Low costs?

Transplantation with bone plugs from the patient's own body incur no production costs. It saves money and has advantages for health care finances, the hospital and the patient.

Fusion with plugs has a stable and perfect consolidation in the vertebral column and the fusion segmental space is stronger on both sides than before (fig. 2).

Economy

For Health Care

Bone plug transplantations from the patient's own body incur no extra costs.

It helps save money for patients, health care, insurance and hospitals.

- Living bone plugs
- Small plugs (about 5–6 cm^3)
- Effective

Comment

Several patients who had already had an operation on the lumbar column and were still suffering back pains consulted the author.

Causes of strong back pain were due to instrumentation with foreign materials (fig. 3–5; metal allergy). The author normally referred the patients back to the surgeon who had originally performed the operation.

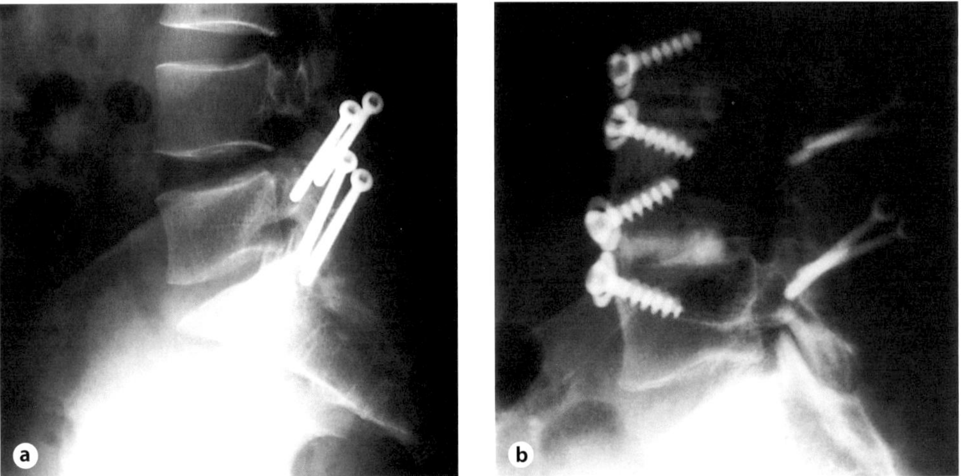

Fig. 3. a Posterior fixation of the screws. **b** Ventral and dorsal fixation of the screws.

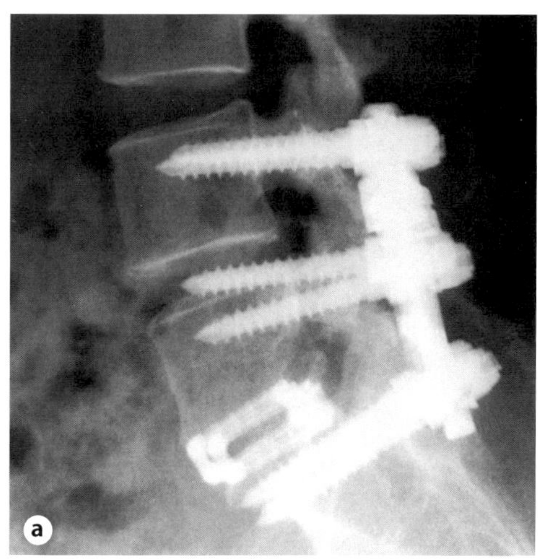

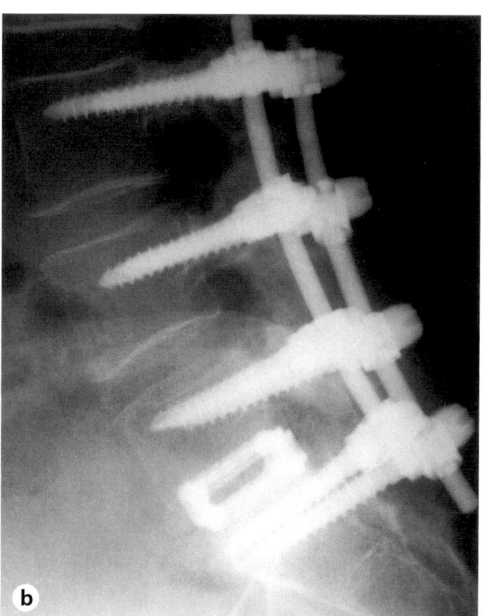

Fig. 4. Plate, screw and cage.

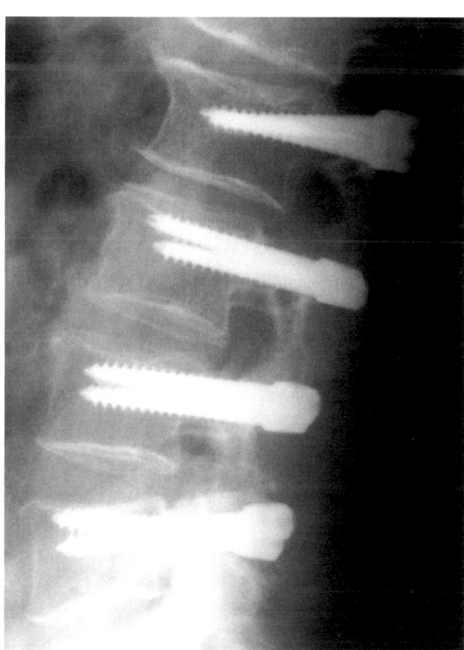

Fig. 5. Several vertebral column fixations.

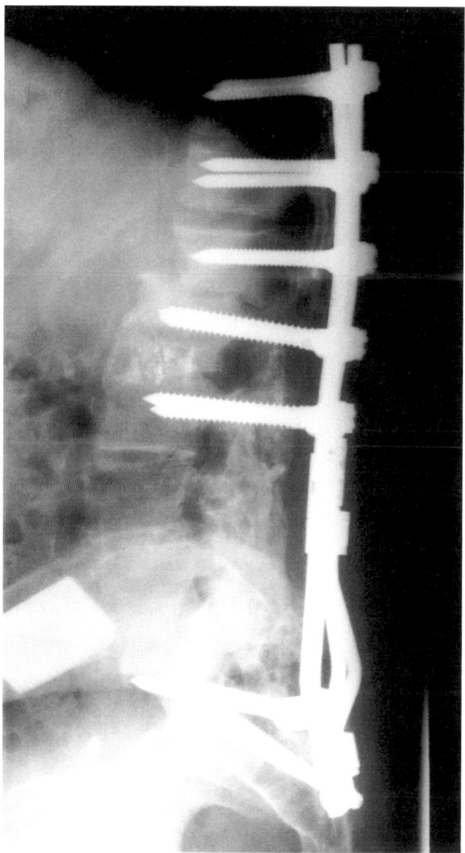

Fig. 6. Several vertebral body fixations.

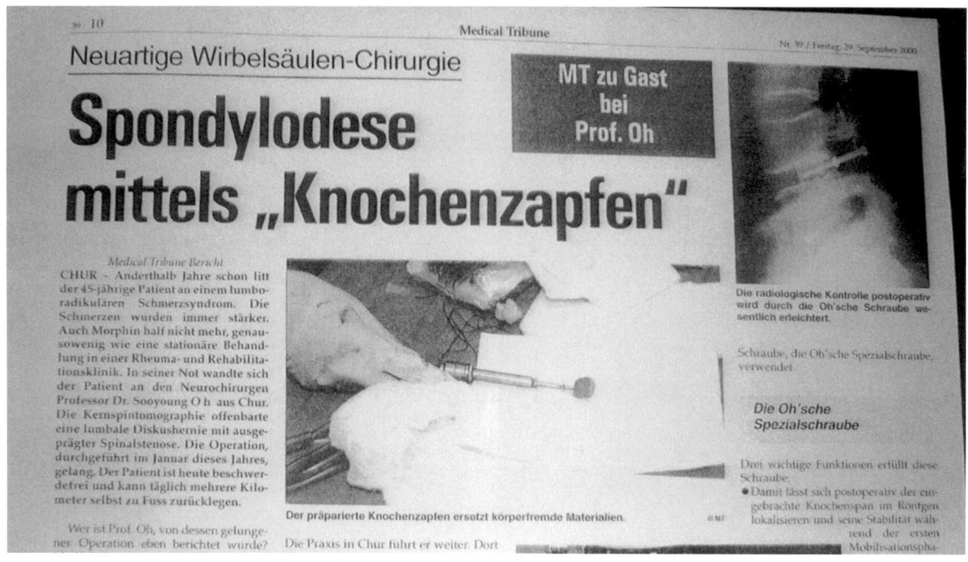

Medical Tribune

Neuartige Wirbelsäulen-Chirurgie

MT zu Gast bei Prof. Oh

Spondylodese mittels „Knochenzapfen"

Medical Tribune Bericht

CHUR – Anderthalb Jahre schon litt der 45-jährige Patient an einem lumboradikulären Schmerzsyndrom. Die Schmerzen wurden immer stärker. Auch Morphin half nicht mehr, genausowenig wie eine stationäre Behandlung in einer Rheuma- und Rehabilitationsklinik. In seiner Not wandte sich der Patient an den Neurochirurgen Professor Dr. Sooyoung O h aus Chur. Die Kernspintomographie offenbarte eine lumbale Diskushernie mit ausgeprägter Spinalstenose. Die Operation, durchgeführt im Januar dieses Jahres, gelang. Der Patient ist heute beschwerdefrei und kann täglich mehrere Kilometer selbst zu Fuss zurücklegen.

Wer ist Prof. Oh, von dessen gelungener Operation eben berichtet wurde?

Der präparierte Knochenzapfen ersetzt körperfremde Materialien.

Die Praxis in Chur führt er weiter. Dort

Die radiologische Kontrolle postoperativ wird durch die Oh'sche Schraube wesentlich erleichtert.

Schraube, die Oh'sche Spezialschraube, verwendet.

Die Oh'sche Spezialschraube

Drei wichtige Funktionen erfüllt diese Schraube:

- Damit lässt sich postoperativ der eingebrachte Knochenspan im Röntgen lokalisieren und seine Stabilität während der ersten Mobilisationspha-

Fig. 7. *Medical Tribune* reports: bone plug fusion is economical.

Several times, the author was also able to remove the posterior screw (fig. 3a), but as shown in figure 3b, it was impossible to remove the ventral screw. In the case depicted in figure 4a, b, of the screw, plate and cage, only the screw and plate were removed; the cage is still in place (fig. 5, 6).

In cases where a patient had so much foreign materials in his body as shown in the case in figure 5, the author referred the patient back to the family doctor or surgeon.

Prof. Dr. med. S. Oh
Facharzt für Neurochirurgie FMH
Grabenstrasse 47
CH 7000 Chur / Switzerland
Tel *41-81 – 252 28 30
Fax *41 – 81 – 252 28 31

Mr.
Georg J. Kaptain, M.D.
Department of Neurosurgery
Health Sciences Center
Box 212
University. of Virginia
Charlottesville, Virginia 22908
USA

July. 25. 2'000

Dear Dr. Kaptain

I was very interested in reading your publication from the Journal of Neurosurgery (Spine) about complications.
My meaning is that *fusion* and *fixation* is not the same (very important).
For example a fracture of a bone must be fixed with plates and screws for reaching fusion, because the material will be removed later (osteosynthese). This is a fusion between bone and bone.
The contrary is fixation: bone and metal. Bone and metal never will grow together.
I am of the opinion that the treatments of the lumbar spine was not correct, because the patients became fixation and **no fusion.**

Enclosed this letter you will find my research paper about lumbar fusion (**autologus bone and bone**). My technique is a fusion *bone-bone*. I am thoroughly convinced that in the near future my method will have a great success, because it is very digestible for patients and also for health-care: no high costs because no metal.
The 67 patients in your report (complications) seems to me very doubtful, why so many complications happened?

I would be very grateful if I would get your feedback.
I am looking forward to hearing from you.

Sincerely,

Sooyoung Oh, M.D.

Encl.: Bone plugs fusion for treatment of lumbar Spondylolisthesis

Fig. 8. Discussion about instrumentation surgery (the author never received an answer to this letter).

J Neurosurg (Spine 1) 93:45–52, 2000

Complications of posterior lumbar interbody fusion when using a titanium threaded cage device

W. Jeffrey Elias, M.D., Nathan E. Simmons, M.D., George J. Kaptain, M.D., James B. Chadduck, M.D., and Richard Whitehill, M.D.

Departments of Neurosurgery and Orthopedic Surgery, University of Virginia Health Sciences Center, Charlottesville; and Winchester Neurosurgical Consultants, Winchester, Virginia

Object. The authors reviewed their series of patients to quantify clinical and radiographic complications in those who underwent a posterior lumbar interbody fusion (PLIF) procedure in which a threaded interbody cage (TIC) was implanted.

Methods. Sixty-seven patients underwent a posterior lumbar interbody fusion procedure in which a TIC was used. The authors excluded patients who underwent procedures in which other instrumentation was used or a nondorsal approach was performed. Fifteen percent of the cases (10 patients) were complicated by laceration of the dura. In three cases, bilateral implantation could not be performed. The average blood loss was 670 ml for all cases, and blood transfusion was required in 25% of the cases (17 patients). The rate of minor wound complication was 4.5% (three patients). One patient died. The average period of hospitalization was 4.25 days.

Twenty-eight patients (42%) experienced significant low-back pain 3 months postoperatively, and in 10 (15%) of these cases it persisted beyond 1 year. In 10 patients postoperative radiculopathy was demonstrated, and magnetic resonance imaging revealed epidural fibrosis in six patients, arachnoiditis in one, and a recurrent disc herniation in one. One patient incurred a permanent motor deficit with sexual dysfunction. Pseudarthrosis was suggested radiographically with evidence of motion on lateral flexion–extension radiographs (10 cases), lucencies around the implants (seven cases), and posterior migration of the cage (two cases).

Additional procedures (in 14 patients) consisted primarily of transverse process fusion with pedicle screw and plate augmentation for persistent back pain and radiographically demonstrated signs of spinal instability. In two patients with radiculopathy, migration of the TIC required that it be removed. Graft material that extruded from one implant necessitated its removal. In one patient scarectomy was performed.

Conclusions. Our high incidence of TIC-related complications in PLIF is inconsistent with that reported in previous studies.

Fig. 9. Treated interbody cage complications.

For a discussion about instrumentation surgery see figure 8. The abstract from an article on treated interbody cage complications is shown in figure 9, and figure 10 depicts cage dislocations following attempted fixation of L4–5 for grade I spondylolisthesis.

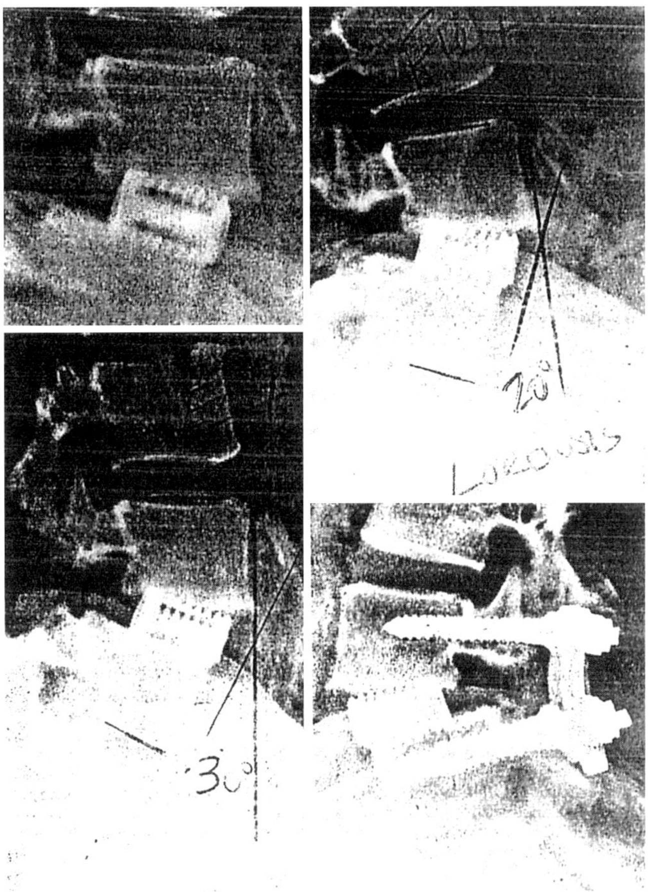

Fig. 10. Cage dislocations (expensive care).

Steps Towards Recognition

- One of the largest Swiss insurance companies, Helsana, recognized Oh's fusion method in March 2001 (letter, fig. 11).
- Official support by Swiss insurance (Santésuisse) company for state acknowledgement in February 2003 (letter, fig. 12).
- More than 60 patients came together to form an action group for recognition of the procedure by state government healthcare, June 2003 (see letter, fig.13).
- In October 2003, the Federal Health Office confirmed its acknowledgement of Oh's fusion procedure and decided that the health insurance would have to take on the cost for the treatment from 01.01.2004 (see letter, fig. 14).

Helsana Versicherungen AG

Managed Care
Talacker 42
8001 Zürich

www.helsana.ch

Zuständig:
Direktwahl

HELSANA

Prof. Dr. med. S. Oh
per FAX Nr. 081 252 28 31

21. März 2001

Tarifvorschläge

Sehr geehrter Herr Prof. Oh

Besten Dank für Ihr Schreiben vom 5. März 2001. Da ich neu die Regionenverantwortlichkeit für die Region Ostschweiz von Peter Indra übernommen habe, bitte ich Sie, inskünftige Fragen an mich zu richten.

Mit Ihren Vorschlägen sind wir grundsätzlich einverstanden. Gerne akzeptieren wir die nachfolgenden Tarife:

1.	Cerivcale OH mit Spondylodese 1 Etage	HP	13'000.--	P	15'000.--
2.	idem auf 2 Etagen	HP	14'000.--	P	17'000.--
3.	LDH 1 Etage	HP	13'000.--	P	14'000.--
4.	LDH mehrere Etagen oder Rezidiv	HP	15'000.--	P	17'000.--
5.	Lumbale Stenose und LDH	HP	16'000.--	P	18'000.--
6.	Oh'sche Fusion lumbal	HP	18'000.--	P	21'000.--
7.	Schraubenentfernung nach Oh's Op	HP	5'000.--	P	7'000.--

Den ausgearbeiteten Vertrag werden Sie in den nächsten Tagen erhalten.

Leider können wir Ihrem Wunsch, dass der Vertrag nur auf Ihre Person lautet und nicht auf den Namen der Klinik, nicht entsprechen. Wir sind jedoch gerne bereit, mit der Klinik "Marienfried" in Niederuzwil sowie der "Neurochirurgischen Klinik" an der Universität Bern den gleichen Vertrag abzuschliessen. Der Vertrag wird auf die jeweils betroffene Klinik lauten und von Ihnen sowie der Klinikdirektion unterschrieben werden müssen.

Ich freue mich auf eine angenehme Zusammenarbeit und stehe Ihnen für Fragen gerne zur Verfügung.

Mit freundlichen Grüssen
Helsana Versicherungen AG

Verantwortlicher Leistungseinkauf Region Ost

Fig. 11. Letter from Helsana, one of the largest Swiss insurance companies. Costs shown include hospital stay and full treatment.

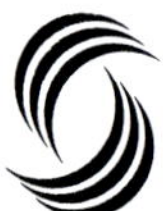

santésuisse | Die Schweizer Krankenversicherer
Les assureurs-maladie suisses
Gli assicuratori malattia svizzeri

Römerstrasse 20
Postfach
CH-4502 Solothurn
Tel. 032 625 41 41
Fax 032 625 41 51
mail@santesuisse.ch
www.santesuisse.ch

Herrn
Prof. Dr. med. S. Oh
Grabenstrasse 47
7000 Chur

Für Rückfragen:
Julian Schilling
Direktwahl: **032 625 42 50**
E-Mail: **julian.schilling@santesuisse.ch**

Solothurn, 24. Februar 2003

Spondylodese

Sehr geehrter Herr Professor Oh

Eine gute Nachricht: santésuisse hat, wie bereits mitgeteilt, Ende 2002 nach Rücksprache mit den beteiligten Versicherern beim Bundesamt für Sozialversicherung Antrag um Abklärung der Umstrittenheit der Spondylodese mittels Knochentransplantat gestellt. Dies mit einer Stellungnahme im positiven Sinne und mit der Anfrage auf das vereinfachte Verfahren erfolgt ist.

Für uns ist die Sache damit vorläufig abgeschlossen. In der Beilage retournieren wir Ihnen Ihre Unterlagen zu unserer Entlastung.

Mit freundlichen Grüssen und den besten Wünschen

santésuisse
Beauftragter für Qualitätssicherung

PD Dr. med. Julian Schilling

Fig. 12. Official supporting letter from Santésuisse.

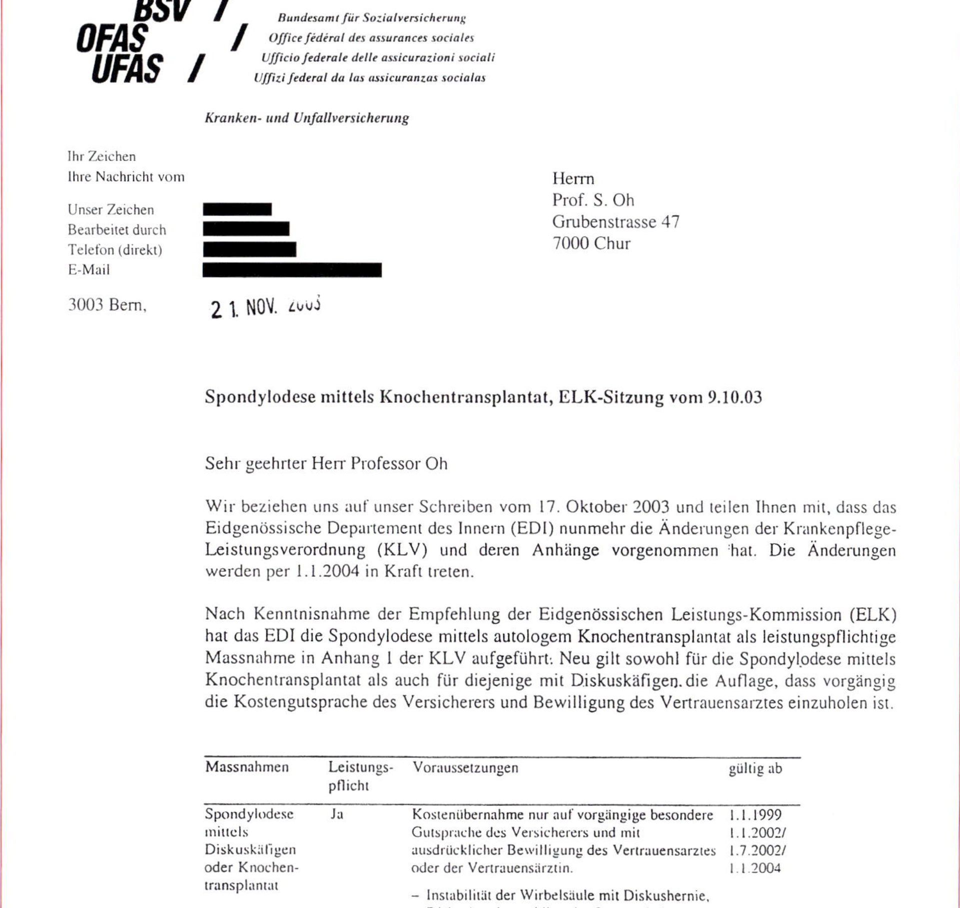

BSV / OFAS / UFAS /

Bundesamt für Sozialversicherung
Office fédéral des assurances sociales
Ufficio federale delle assicurazioni sociali
Uffizi federal da las assicuranzas socialas

Kranken- und Unfallversicherung

Ihr Zeichen
Ihre Nachricht vom

Unser Zeichen [redacted]
Bearbeitet durch [redacted]
Telefon (direkt) [redacted]
E-Mail [redacted]

3003 Bern, 21. NOV. 2003

Herrn
Prof. S. Oh
Grubenstrasse 47
7000 Chur

Spondylodese mittels Knochentransplantat, ELK-Sitzung vom 9.10.03

Sehr geehrter Herr Professor Oh

Wir beziehen uns auf unser Schreiben vom 17. Oktober 2003 und teilen Ihnen mit, dass das Eidgenössische Departement des Innern (EDI) nunmehr die Änderungen der Krankenpflege-Leistungsverordnung (KLV) und deren Anhänge vorgenommen hat. Die Änderungen werden per 1.1.2004 in Kraft treten.

Nach Kenntnisnahme der Empfehlung der Eidgenössischen Leistungs-Kommission (ELK) hat das EDI die Spondylodese mittels autologem Knochentransplantat als leistungspflichtige Massnahme in Anhang 1 der KLV aufgeführt. Neu gilt sowohl für die Spondylodese mittels Knochentransplantat als auch für diejenige mit Diskuskäfigen die Auflage, dass vorgängig die Kostengutsprache des Versicherers und Bewilligung des Vertrauensarztes einzuholen ist.

Massnahmen	Leistungspflicht	Voraussetzungen	gültig ab
Spondylodese mittels Diskuskäfigen oder Knochentransplantat	Ja	Kostenübernahme nur auf vorgängige besondere Gutsprache des Versicherers und mit ausdrücklicher Bewilligung des Vertrauensarztes oder der Vertrauensärztin. – Instabilität der Wirbelsäule mit Diskushernie, Diskushernienrezidiv oder Stenose bei Patienten mit therapieresistenten invalidisierenden spondylogenen oder radikulären Schmerzen, bedingt durch klinisch und radiologisch nachgewiesene instabile, degenerative Pathologien der Wirbelsäule. – Nach Misserfolg einer hinteren Spondylodese mit Pedikelschraubensystem.	1.1.1999 1.1.2002/ 1.7.2002/ 1.1.2004

Wir hoffen, Ihnen mit diesen Angaben zu dienen.

Mit freundlichen Grüssen

Krankenversicherung
Medizinische Leistungen

[redacted]

Dr. med. [redacted]

x 031 322 78 80

Kopie an : Schweizerische Gesellschaft für Neurochirurgie, Sekretariat
PD Dr. [redacted] Inselspital, Neurochirurgische Klinik, 3010 Bern

Effingerstrasse 20, 3003 Bern, Telefon 031 322 90 11, Telefax 031 322 78 80
Internet: http://www.bsv.admin.ch

Fig. 13. Letter from the Swiss federal government of social security confirming the definite acknowledgement of Oh's fusion procedure.

Anatomical Aspects of Lumbar Fusion

For posterior interbody vertebra column fusion, extensive knowledge of the neurotopographical anatomy is required from the surgeon.

Various congenital abnormalities exist, e.g. spondylosis and spondylolisthesis, but no correlation has been found yet for any related instability.

Vertebral Column

Male and female, young and old patients show very variable contours of the vertebral column, especially concerning the stenotic reactions which occur after disc surgery.

- Topographical situations are shown in figure 14a, b.
- Knowledge of the nerve root, nerve canal, facet joint and intervertebral space which is correlated is important for the fusion procedure.

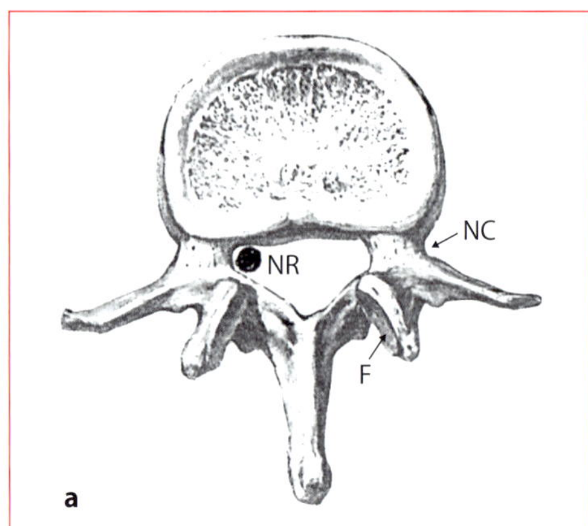

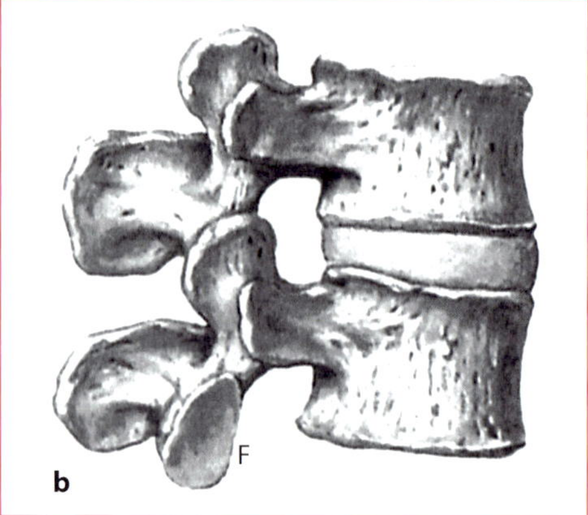

Fig. 14. a, b Vertebral column (A-P lateral). NR = Nerve root; NC = nerve canal; F = facet joint.

Intervertebral Space

The segmental interbody space is occupied mostly by discus material (nucleus pulposus) (fig. 15).

If the disc is damaged, a compression of the nerve roots is most likely present. With unstable facet joints instability and deformation of intervertebral space occur. On the other hand, a wide vertebral space is rarely observed (fig. 16a). Where there is a space of more than 14 mm, Oh's fusion procedure is not recommended from a technical standpoint, as there are difficulties and a danger of damage to the nerve roots during insertion of the plugs. With intervertebral body stenosis (fig. 16b), the handling for fusion is maneuverable and easier than with a wide intervertebral space (fig. 16a, b).

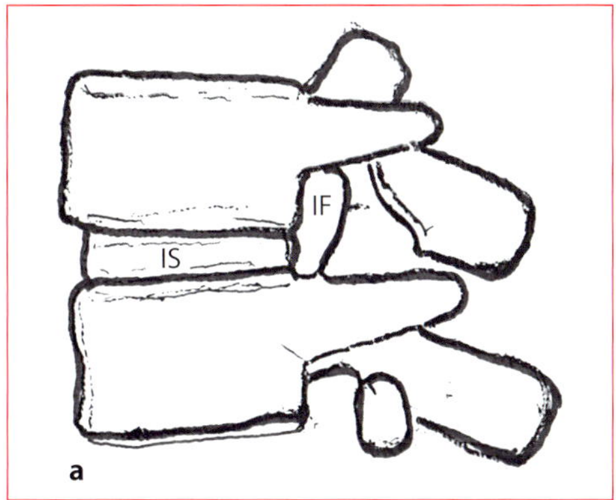

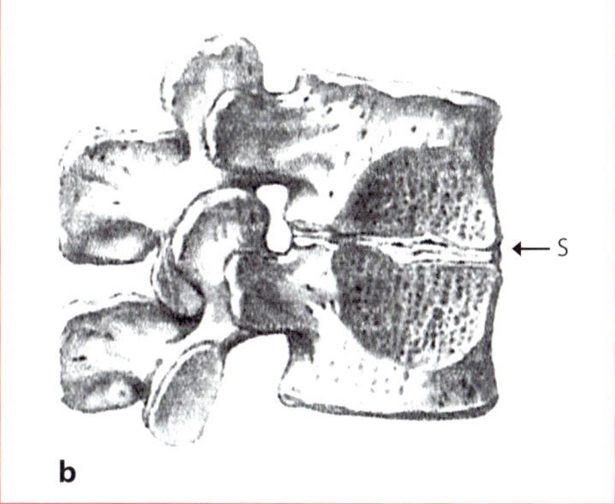

Fig. 15. a, b Lateral view: intervertebral space. IS = Intervertebral space; IF = intervertebral foramen; S = stenosis.

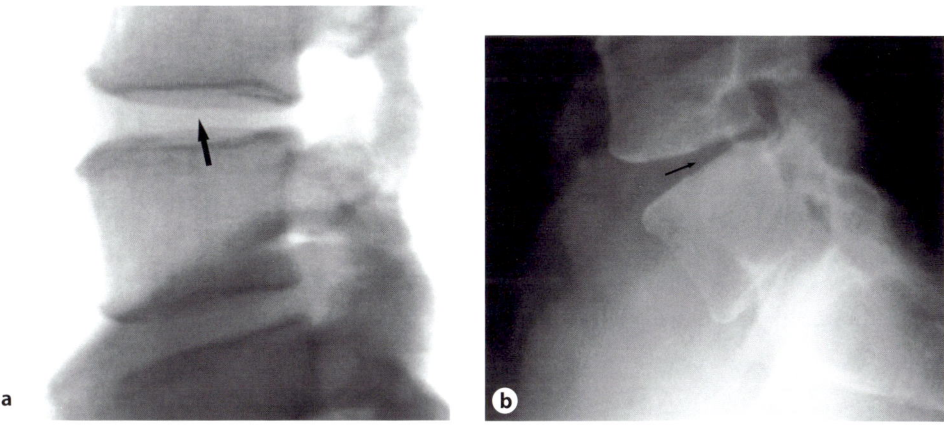

Fig. 16. a Large intervertebral space. **b** Narrow intervertebral space.

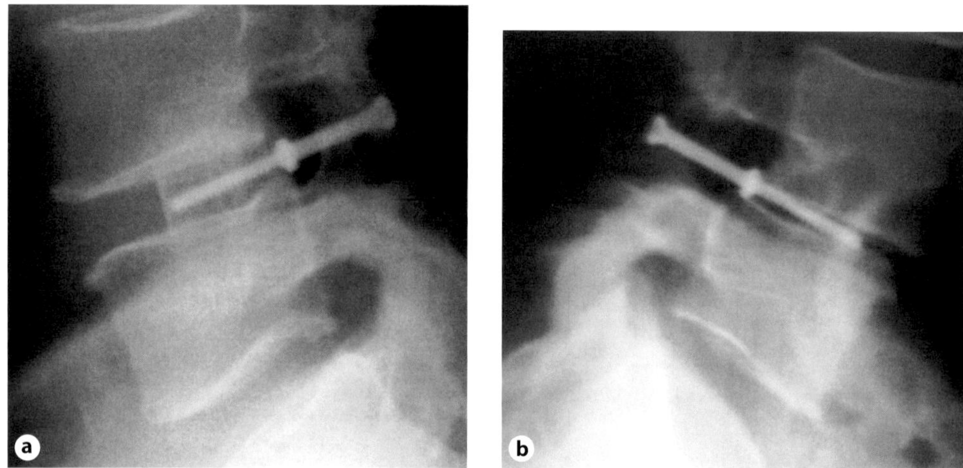

Fig 17. a Large interspace fusion. **b** Narrow interspace fusion.

Comment

The drill size has to be correlated to the interbody space, and the right choice is important (fig. 17). From clinical experience, the narrowest interbody space measured was 5 mm while the largest was 14 mm, i.e. an average of 10 mm. A fusion procedure where the intervertebral space is wider than 14 mm is not possible.

For performing compact fusion, the plugs usually have to be 4 mm bigger than the drilled interbody space hole (see table 3).

In a fusion procedure where the interbody space is wider than 14 mm, making an intervertebral drill hole is not advisable because the process of plug insertion is dangerous due to potential damaging of the nerve roots.

Nerve Roots Correlation

(Lumbo-Sacral Area)

Nerve root L5 is normally located on segmental level L4/5 (fig. 18–23). Congenital malformation of lumbo-sacralization appears in the same position, although interspace mobility is different.

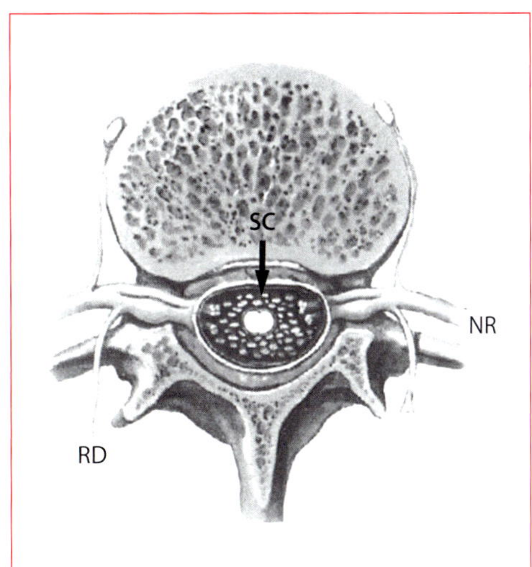

Fig. 18. Nerve root canal. SC = Spine canal; NR = nerve root; RD = ramus dorsalis.

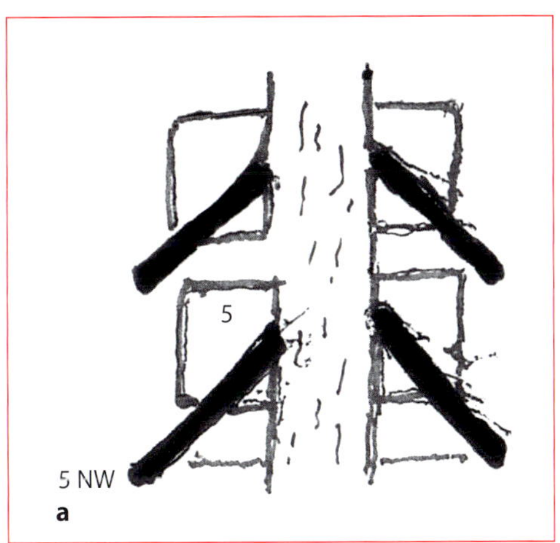

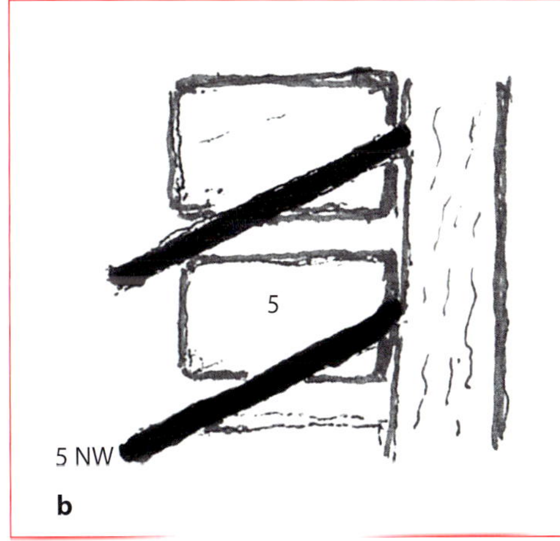

Fig. 19. A-P view (**a**) nerve root innervations on the segmental level. Lateral view (**b**). Level L4/5 innervated L5 nerve root.

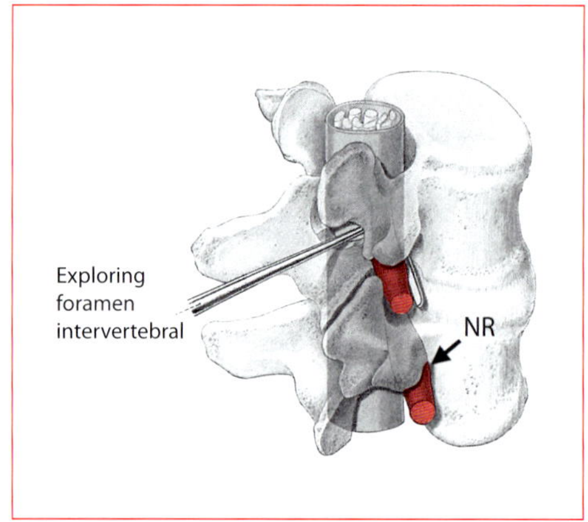

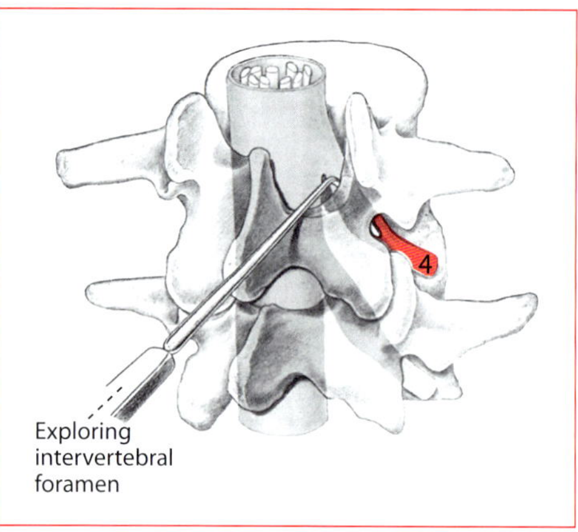

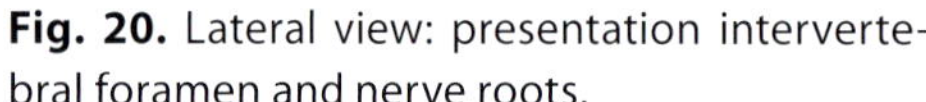

Fig. 20. Lateral view: presentation intervertebral foramen and nerve roots.

Fig. 21. Posterior view: intervertebral. Foramen and dorsal to the nerve root through the foramina intervertebralia.

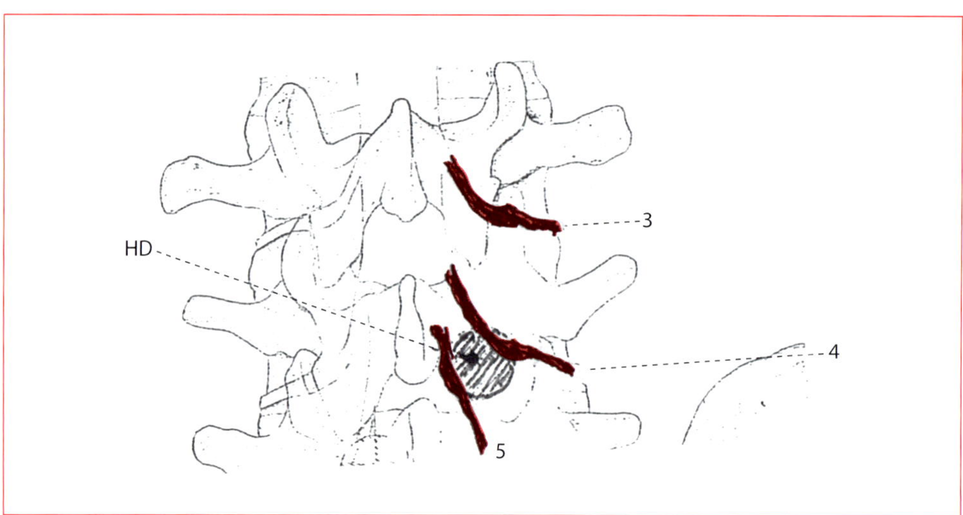

Fig. 22. Anatomical topographical presentation of lumbar nerve roots. Relationship of the nerve roots to the intervertebral disc space and canal. HD = Herniated disc.

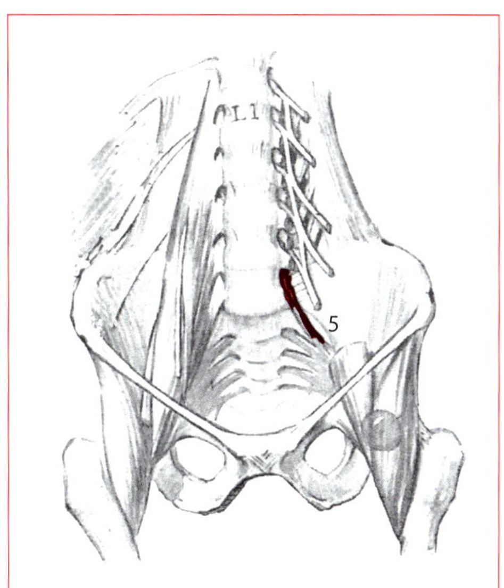

Fig. 23. Illustration of sacral nerve roots.

Important aspects of the lateral part of the interbody space are that the nerve root canal is located there (fig. 16). Facet joint instability produces nerve root syndrome.

For example, a herniated disc may compress the nerve root L4 laterally and the L5 nerve root medially (fig. 22, 23).

Clinical Consideration of Instability

Instability may have different causes. Mostly, spondylolisthesis with instable joints was found. Post disc surgery with micro-instability is not rare and commends surgical treatment for better results. Especially united fusion methods contrast considerably with fixation methods.

Inducement of Instability

- Spondylosis
- Spondylolisthesis
- Instability following herniated disc surgery
- Traumatics
- Unknown
- Type of instabilities:
  - Mono segmental
  - Double segmental

Spondylosis

- Radiological pictures show the separation of the pars interarticulares of the vertebral arch (fig. 24).
- In 1855, Robert describes the first congenital form.
- Statistics show that it affects 4.5% of children and 6% of adults.
- Mostly ill patients with long-term recurrent back pain.

While protruded discs are the common cause of nerve root compression in the middle years, the fourth and fifth decades are marked by dehydration and collapse of the nucleus and bulging in all directions of the annulus, which becomes calcified or ossified; new bone forms along the adjacent vertebral margins, creating lips or spurs.

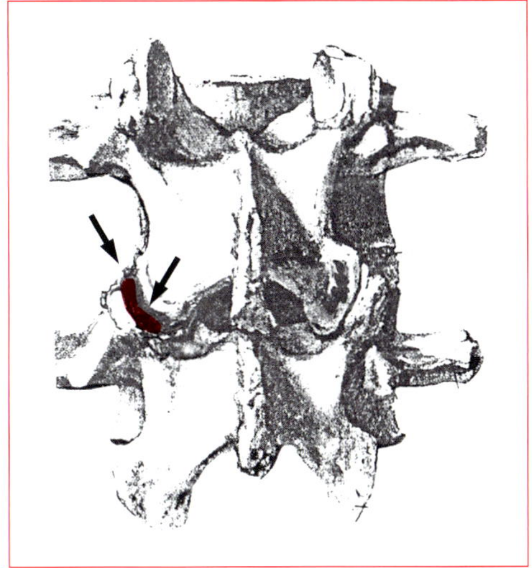

Fig. 24. Separation of the facet joint left (spondylosis).

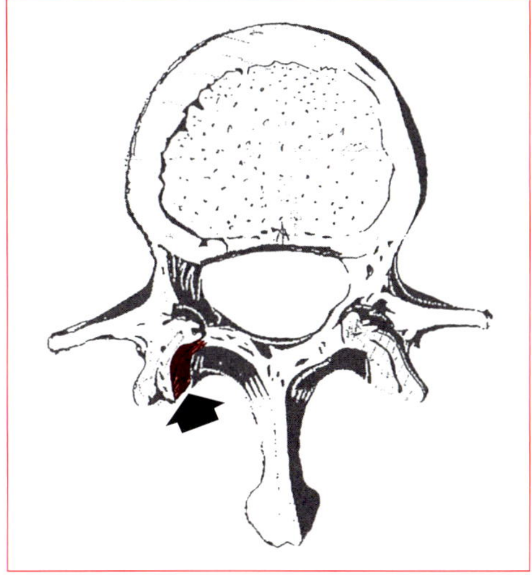

Fig. 25. Anteroposterior view of spondylosis.

With collapse of the disc, there is subluxation of the corresponding intervertebral joints (fig. 25) and narrowing of the intervertebral foramina, which may be further compromised by osteophytic formation at the articular processes (fig. 26).

The syndrome may be indistinguishable from that of a ruptured intervertebral disc, although the pain is usually less severe than sciatic pain if there is disc herniation and it is less likely to be exacerbated by coughing or sneezing. Dysesthesias with pain may be prominent, and, if several roots are involved, conspicuous muscular weakness, wasting, and reflex changes may be present.

Considerable interest has been focused in recent years on the small but otherwise normal spinal canal that has had its already borderline lumen further compromised by spondylosis (fig. 26).

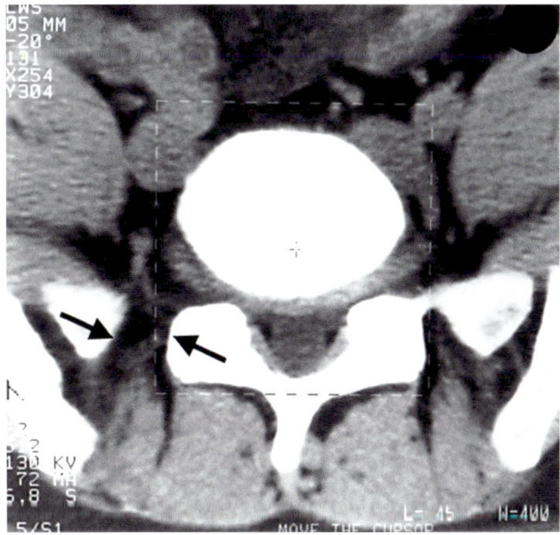

Fig. 26. CT scan reveals separation of the pars interarticularis (spondylosis).

Table 1. Operated patients: 37% were between 40 and 50 years old

Age	Female	Male	Total
30 years	10	9	19
31–40 years	21	10	31
41–50 years	28	23	51
51–60 years	7	9	16
61–70 years	7	4	11
71– years	8	2	10
Total	71	57	138

Spondylolisthesis

Spondylolisthesis occurs in about 5% of the adult population. It is now believed that this malformation is the result of an injury of the facet joint, usually of the fifth lumbar vertebra, which takes place shortly after birth. Cases have been cited that showed that spondylolisthesis can be acquired in later life from repeated stress over a long period of time. The average age of the affected patients being treated is mostly between 40 and 50 years (table 1) which may have a difference of anamnesis of variable spondylolisthesis (see fig. 38–40).

The author's youngest patient was a 15-year-old boy. From this age, the incidence of recognition increases progressively according to the literature; 20% of patients with symptomatic spondylolisthesis are under 20 years old.

Many patients go through life with an asymptomatic spondylolisthesis after trauma, usually extension injuries or those incurred when a strong force is exerted vertically downward upon the spine, but symptoms will appear.

The clinical manifestations are pain and instable deformity. The pain is of two types. Low lumbar pain is thought to be due to instability of the vertebra and the mechanical stresses caused by this mobility. It is accentuated by weight bearing, lifting, and moving, and is relieved by recumbence and rest. It is frequently aggravated by purposeless movements. Often it commences insidiously early in life, gradually increasing in severity, or it may appear suddenly associated with an injury. Leg pain is caused by pressure on the nerve roots of the spinal canal and is less common than backache. Various authors have pointed out that the pain results from nerve root compression from degenerative and proliferative changes in the pseudo-arthrosis and rarely from associated disc herniation.

At the level of the stair-like deformity between the vertebrae, the double-layer displacement makes a double bend and is often densely adherent, but in most instances the cauda equina is not actually compressed. If it is compressed, bladder function is disturbed.

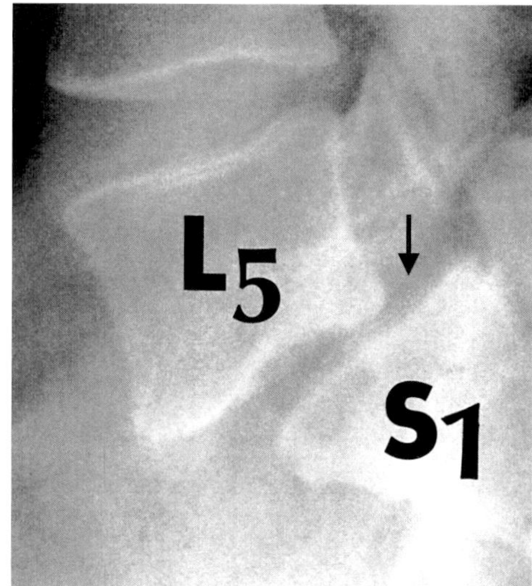

Fig. 27. Spondylolisthesis L5/S1.

On examination, a deformity of the back may not be noticed, but in severe cases there is a mono-type change in the displaced facet ligament of the tips of the spines at the lumbosacral level. Characteristically, the pelvis is rotated backward so that the sacrum becomes more dorsal in an attempt to realign the weight of the body for more adequate support. In extreme cases, the hips and knees will be slightly flexed, the trunk tilted forward, and some scoliosis may be present. In extremely severe deformities, the trunk cannot be held erect over the legs and settles down into the pelvis so that the lower ribs touch the iliac crest and folds appear about the waist.

Spondylolisthesis with intact vertebrae can occur. This is usually seen at the L5–S1 level in patients past middle life who have considerable osteoarthritis of the spine and degenerative changes of the articular cartilage of the facets that allow forward displacement and subluxation (fig. 27); it may occur at the L5–S1 level in the elderly from degenerative changes alone. When the vertebral arches are intact, slipping is limited by the impingement of the displaced inferior facet against the body of the vertebra below. The displaced facet thus comes into close contact with the nerve root, which passes toward the pedicle and the intervertebral foramen of the segment below, while the intact isthmus compresses the nerve root posteriorly. In severe deformity of the lumbar sacral region, the entire cauda equina may be compressed by the intact neural arch.

The diagnosis is confirmed only by radiological examination, and oblique view and functional radiological checkups are particularly helpful in revealing defects of the pars interarticularis. If operative intervention is being considered, CT and MRI studies may be useful, particularly a horizontal-beam study made in flexion and extension.

Instability following Herniated Disc Surgery

Postoperative HIVD with Instability

Typical HIVD (as illustrated in fig. 28) is seen in patients which were operated on already 2–4 times for HIVD without improvement.

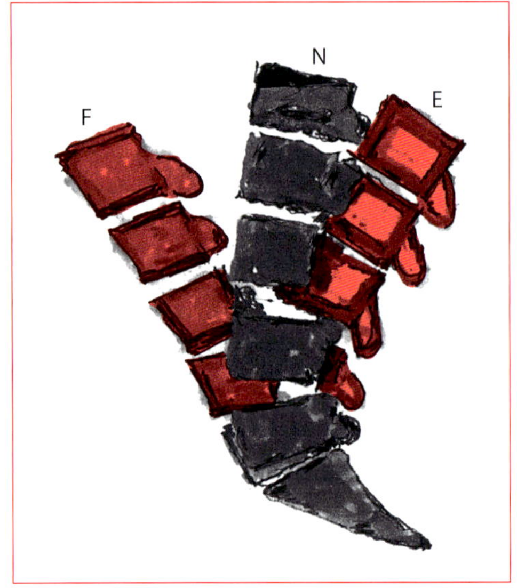

Fig. 28. Functional X-ray movement checking for instability. F = Flexion; N = neutral; E = extension.

- This form is not so rare and is mostly connected with social problems, such as being out of work for a long time, but gives no indication for operation.
- Furthermore, no detection of etiology by general practitioners.
- Postoperative HIVD with micro-instability mostly needs special radiological interventions for the findings (fig. 29–33).
- Special accessories facilitate diagnosis such as simple facet infiltration (see below, fig. 44, 45) and wearing a lumbar corset.
- Some cases have to be carefully re-operated because of severe adhesion in the dura matter and nerve roots.
- Operative technique:
  - Hemilaminectomy
  - Removal of HIVD material
  - Fusion procedure

Functional X-Ray Checking to Find Micro-Instability

It is very important that patients who are suspected to have micro-instability be checked with functional X-rays. Only this method shows a displaced vertebral column, especially by instable listhesis post disc surgery. The X-ray picture shows mostly extension position (fig. 29, 33), i.e. in addition to CT and MRI (fig. 30, 31).

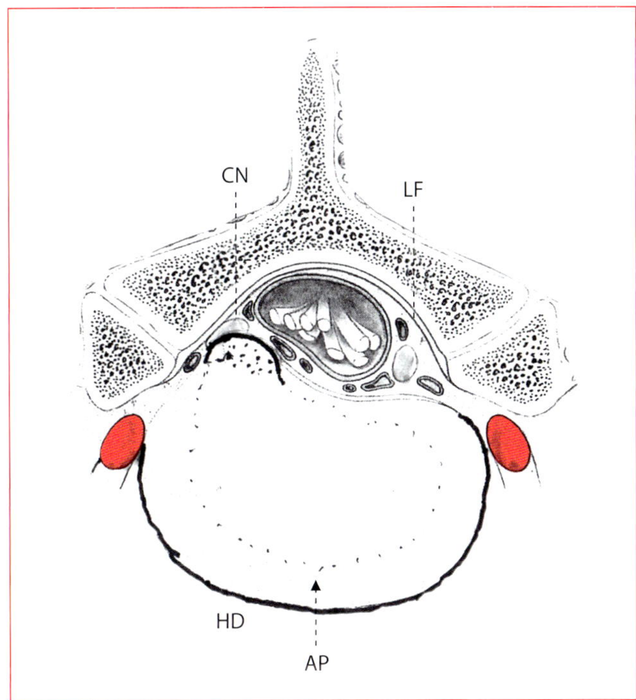

Fig. 29. Lumbar intervertebral herniated disc. CN = Compressed nerve root; LF = ligamentum flavum; HD = herniated disc; AP = anulus pulposis.

Case
M.D., male, born 1951

Anamneses
Operation 1989 (patient was 38 years old) of HIVD on level L4/5.

Second recurred HIVD same level L4/5 was operated again 2 years later.

After both these operations he was complaining about 'only' back pain without any more sciatic pain, occasionally unbearable pains. Strong repeated back pain without neurological deficits, especially no senso-motoric disturbances.

Radiological examination confirmed micro-instability (fig. 33).

Fusion operation was performed in June 1993 (patient was 42 years old at that time) for stabilization with autologous bone plugs (fig. 34).

Postoperative checks were excellent and the patient was free of back pains.

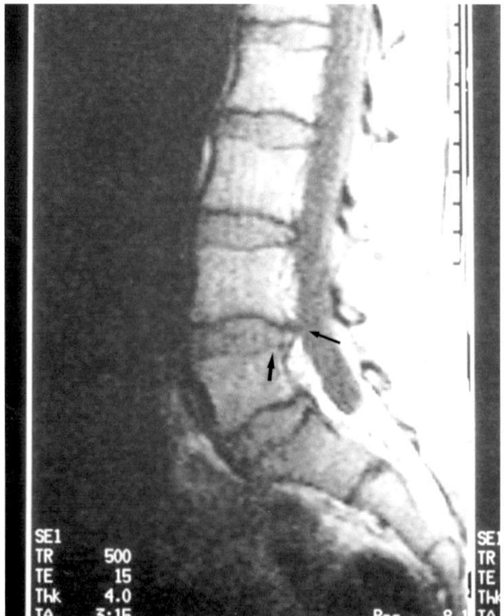

Fig. 30. Spondylolisthesis has caused development of the intervertebral herniated disc on the L4/5 segment.

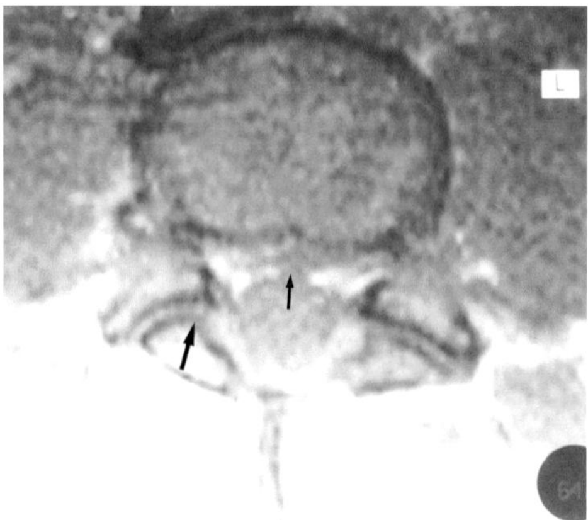

Fig. 31. Mediolateral herniated intervertebral disc on L4/5 with displaced facet joint on both sides.

Comment

The above-mentioned patient was a pilot for an airline before he was ill. After the second operation, he was no longer able to work and was receiving a disability pension. With the treatment of Oh's fusion operation, he feels healthy and is working again full time for an insurance company. He is also president of the action committee for Oh's fusion.

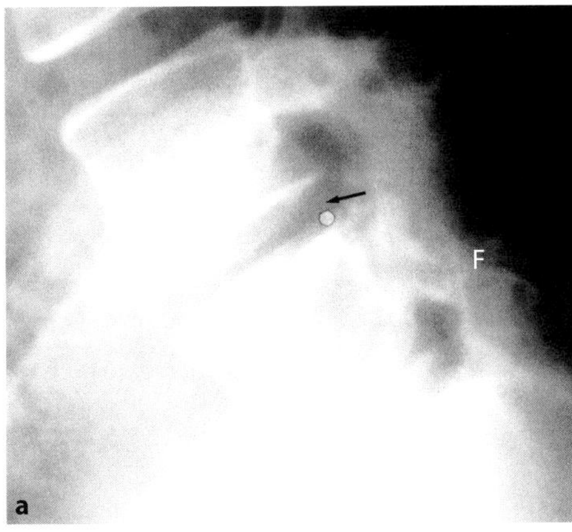

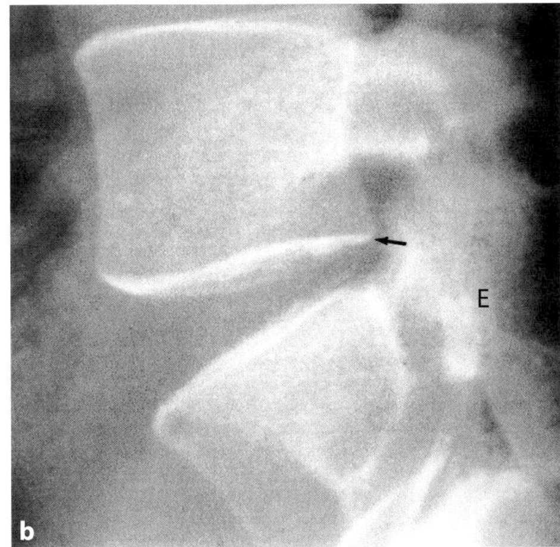

Fig. 32. a, b X-ray showing mostly extension position. F = Flexion; E = extension.

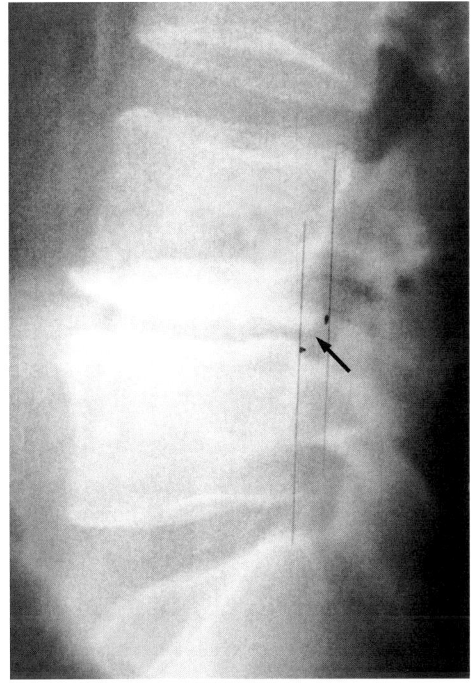

Fig. 33. Functional X-ray in the reclining position shows micro-instability only on layer L4/5.

Traumatic Instability

The evidence shows instability as a result of discus surgery.

Case

A 48-year-old male collided with a tree whilst on a motorcycle. Immediately after the accident he suffered back pains. Functional X-rays showed an approximately 4-mm displacement (fig. 35) by hyperextension. MRI pictures (fig. 36a, b) show listhesis with HIVD L4/5. Subsequent to surgical treatment, stabilizing through Oh's fusion was performed.

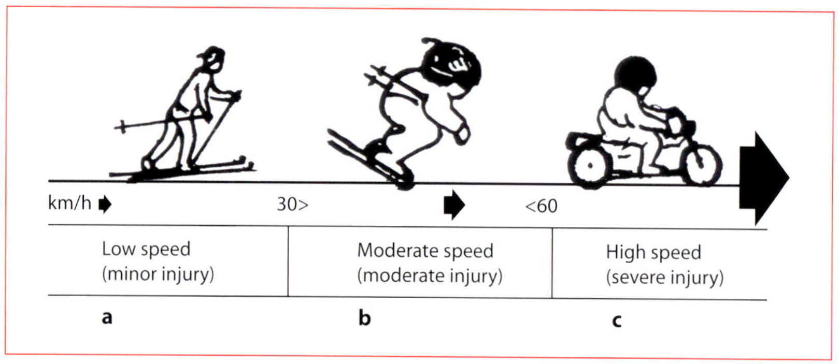

Fig. 34. a–c Speed coordinates to body injury.

Comment
The risk in speed-related accidents correlates in a way that is similar to risks in other forms of locomotion, such as skiing or cycling or motorbike riding where the body of the victim is exposed. The injury of the human body and the speed force are directly related (fig. 34). Average speeds of 60 km/h produce skiing accidents with body injury. Skiing accidents at moderate speeds (30–60 km/h) result in back injury, as shown in many cases observed by the author.

X-ray revealed that the spondylolisthesis may have already existed before.

Unknown

The author reported about 138 cases in 1998. 51 patients complained of back pain, the age of these patients ranged between 40 and 50 years old.

Patients with long-term recurrent pain often had evidence of being involved in accidents. The anamnesis – the health condition before and after an accident – is not always clear.

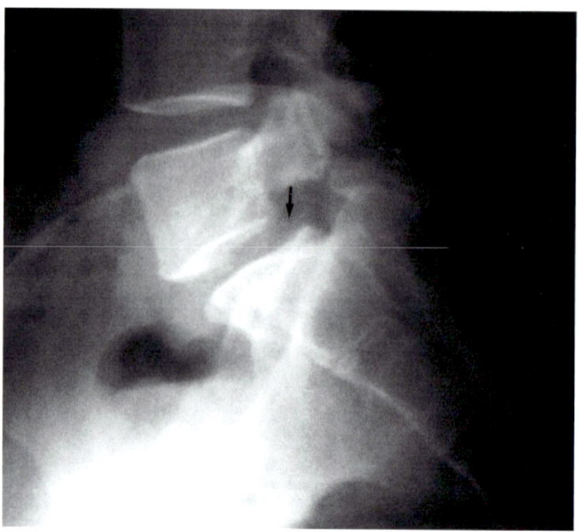

Fig. 35. Displacement probably before accident.

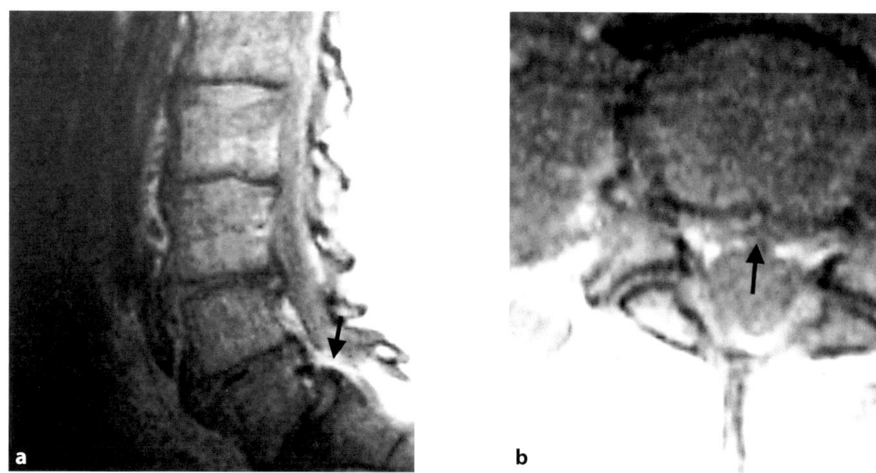

Fig. 36. a Lateral view: unstable spondylolisthesis caused herniated intervertebral disc on L5/S1. **b** Median located herniated disc L5/S1 vertebral arch displaced both sides.

Types of Instability

According to radiological examination, the author classified these as follows:

(1) Type Dorsal 'D'
Single dorsal displacement (fig. 37a).

L5 vertebral column displaced against S1 dorsal position (fig. 38a, b).

(2) 'V' Ventral Type
'L': Step-like deformity, vertebra displaced (L5 ventral to S1) (fig. 37b, 39a, b).

(3) 'DO' Double Level Displaced Form
There are three types of double luxation:

(a) *DD type:* vertebra body L5 is between segment L4/5 and L5/S1 dorsally displaced (fig. 40a, b).

(b) *VD type:* double deformed; vertebra body L5 lies between segments L4/5 and L5/S1 ventrally displaced (fig. 41a, b).

(c) *ST type:* stair-like subluxation:

Double L type L4/5 and L5/S1 built stair-like dorsally displaced (fig. 42a, b).

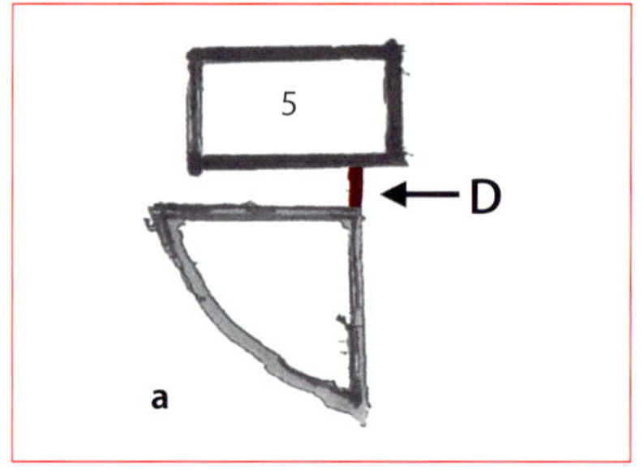

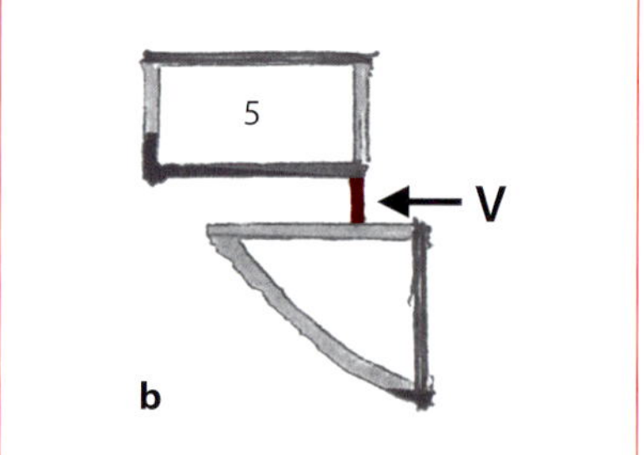

Fig. 37. a Dorsal type. **b** Ventral type.

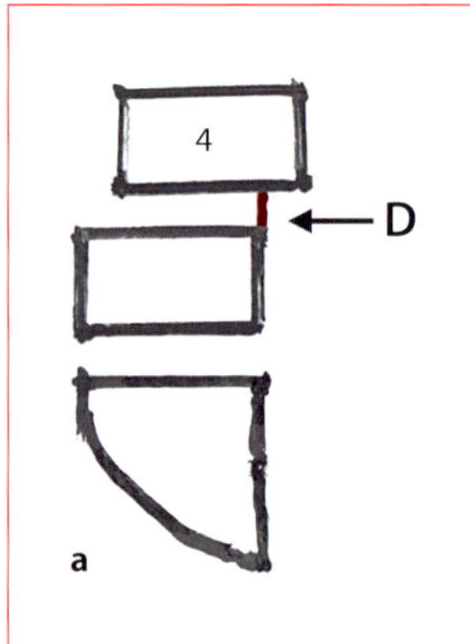

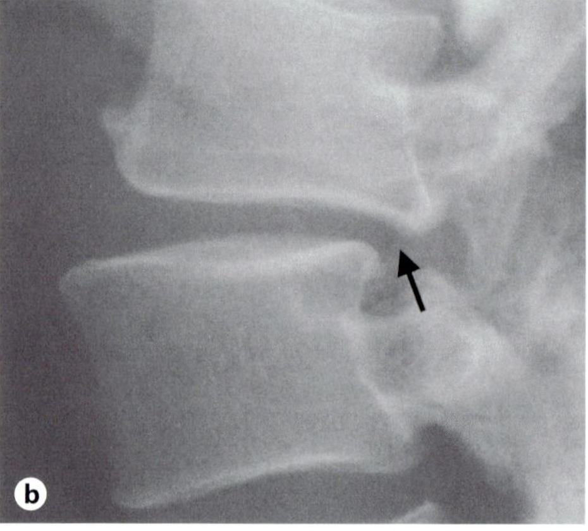

Fig. 38. a, b L4 vertebral subluxated to vertebra L5 dorsal.

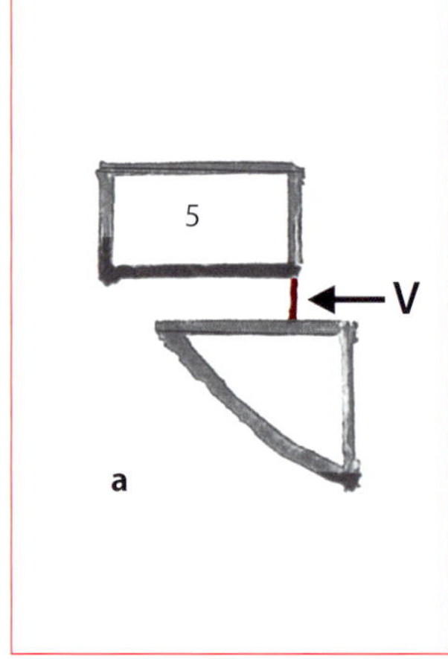

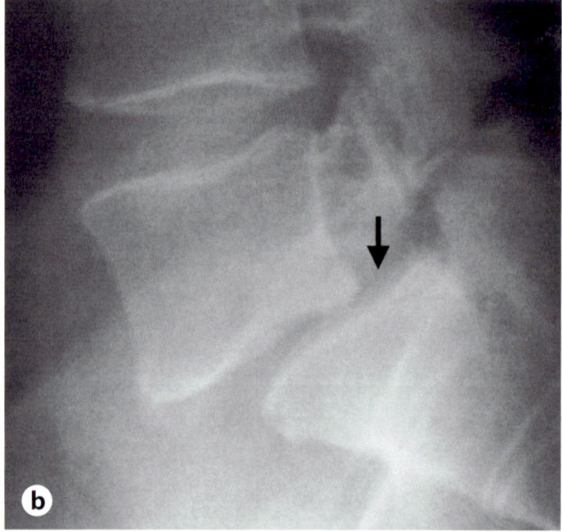

Fig. 39. a, b L5 vertebra is ventrally displaced against S1.

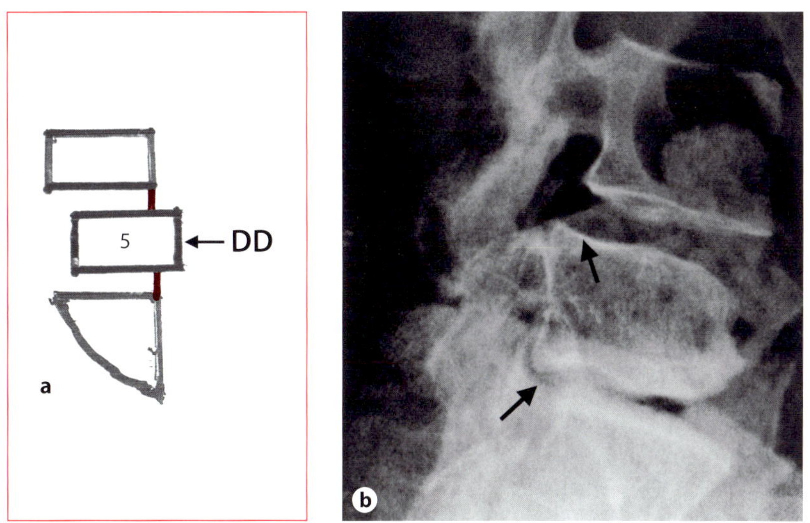

Fig. 40. a, b L5 vertebral column is displaced on L4/5 and L5/S1 dorsal.

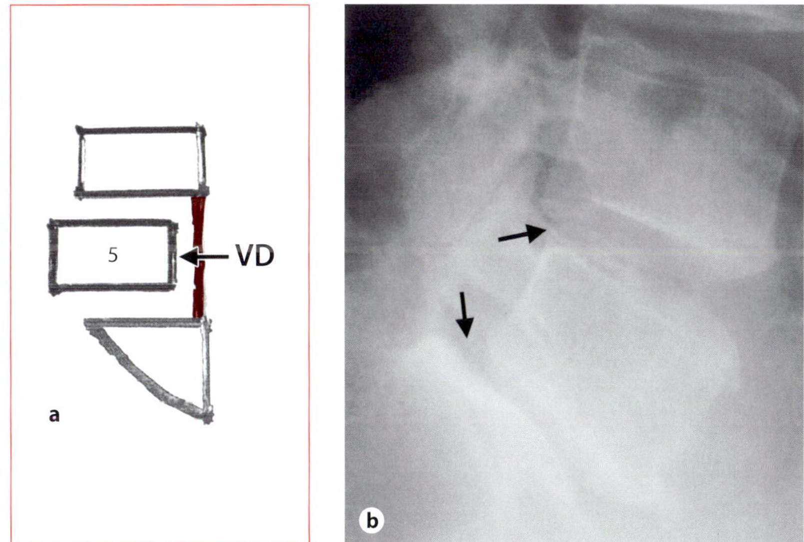

Fig. 41. a, b Double dislocation L4/5 and L5/S1 ventral.

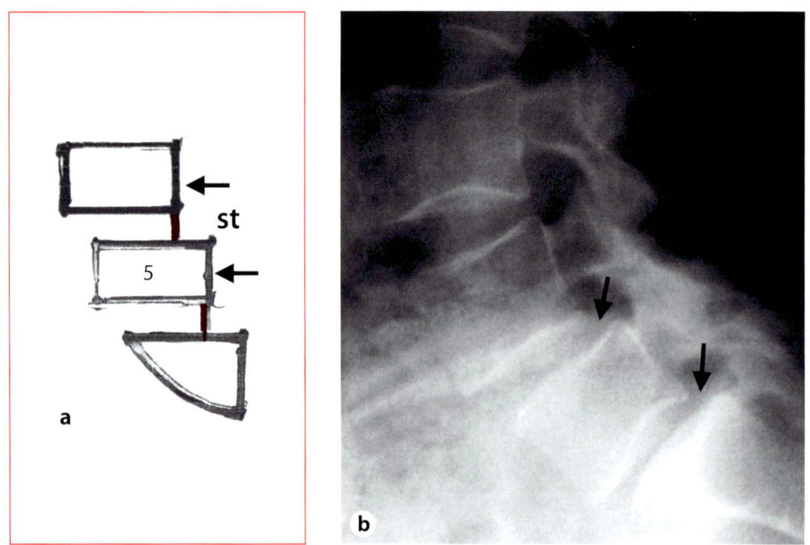

Fig. 42. a, b Stair-like displacement of the double segmental L4/5 and L5/S1.

Indication for Fusion Operation

If the instability is confirmed by X-ray checking, the following measures must be borne in mind:

- Neurological check
- Pain intensity
- Sensory disorder
- Motor weakness
- Bladder dysfunction
- Temporary positive reaction after facet infiltration
- Temporary positive reaction after wearing a lumbar corset

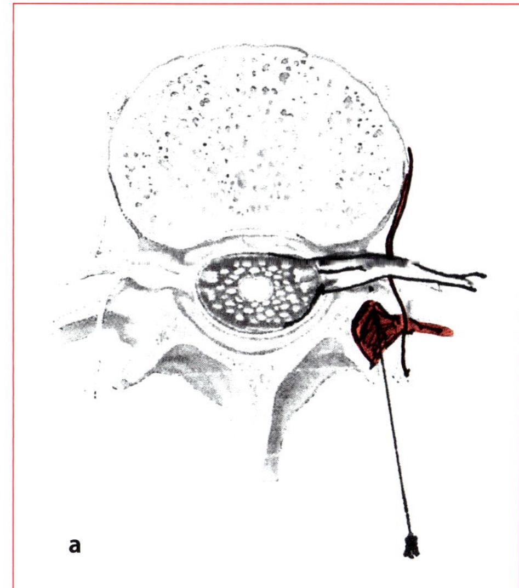

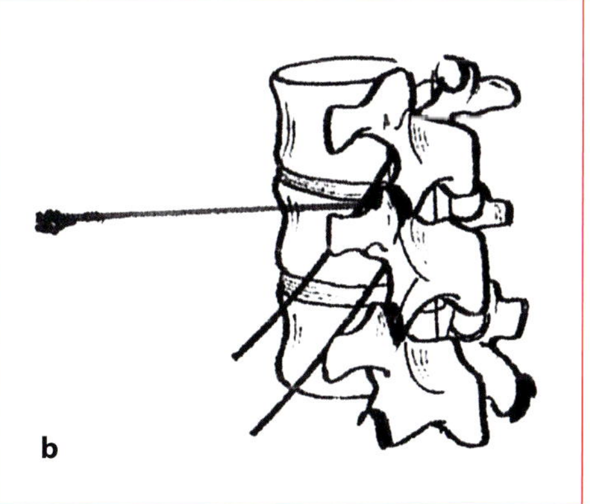

Fig. 43. a, b Facet joint nerve infiltration.

Facet Infiltration or Blockade

- A facet infiltration creates therapeutic and diagnostic options and certainties.
- The reaction of a blockade is locally limited (fig. 43a, b).
- Needle punction must be done under X-ray control because of the danger of damaging nerve roots or dura (fig. 44, 45).
- After injection, the patient has to rest for about 1 h in case of side effects, during this time he has to be observed.
- When the result of infiltration is positive, the procedure can be repeated several times.
- With instability, the facet infiltration only has a diagnostic significance. If the result is temporarily positive, the question of operating may be raised.
- In case of chronic back pain after disc surgery adhesion, repeated periodic blockade is very recommendable.
- In case of spondylosis with back pain only, from the therapeutic point of view, a facet infiltration is also recommendable.

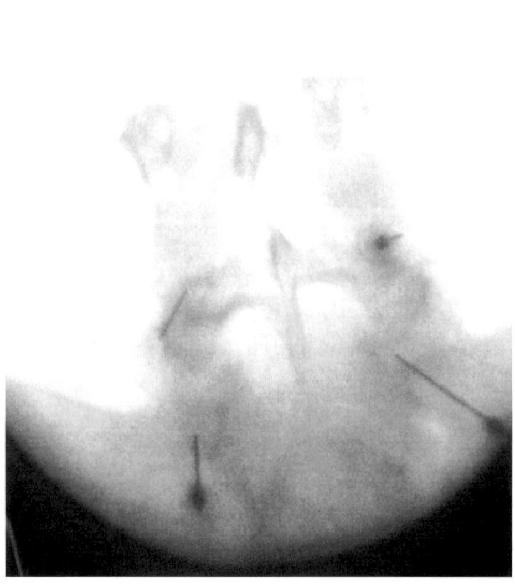

Fig. 44. Needle punction X-ray check of the facet joint in the operation room.

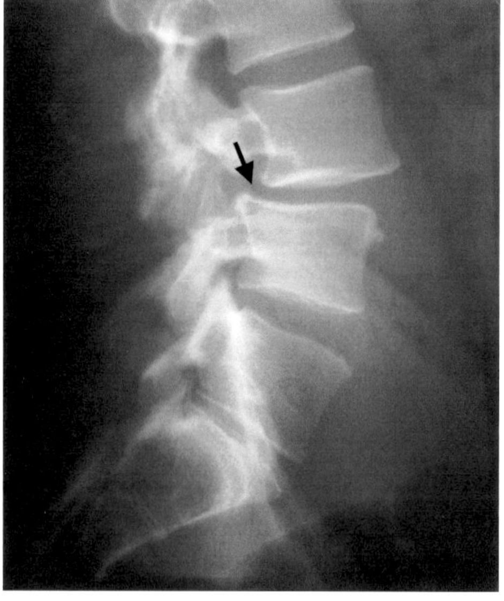

Fig. 45. Instable displacement of L3/4.

Contraindication for Operation

Plugs fusion is a perfect surgical procedure. The following aspects are important for serious indications, and there are four points of contraindication which must be watched for:

(1) No more than 10 mm displacement ventrally or dorsally (fig. 46).

(2) For stable plugs fusion, an interbody distance of at least 20–25 mm is necessary (fig. 47).

(3) High intervertebral spaces must not exceed 14 mm (fig. 48).

(4) Bone plugs with a diameter from 18 mm are necessary; this means 4 mm bigger than the hole. If a diameter of more than 18 mm is used, there is the danger of damage being caused to the nerve root.

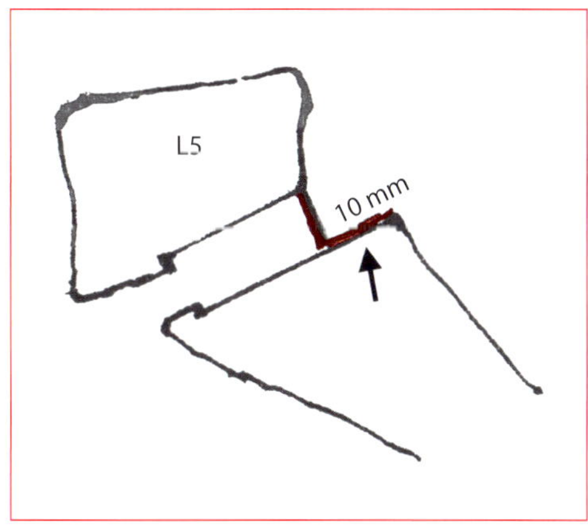

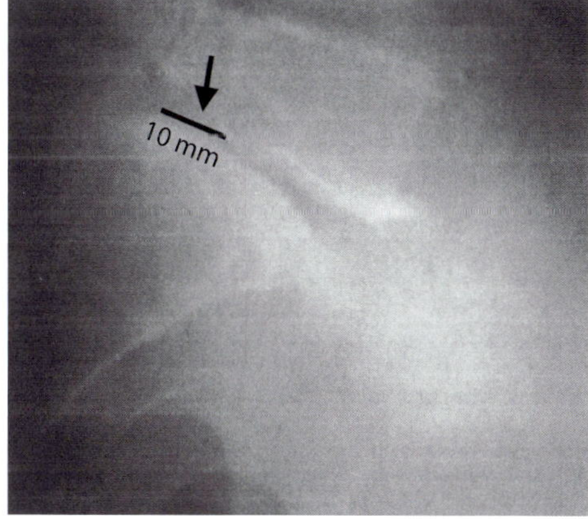

Fig. 46. Not more than 10 mm displacement for stability.

Other Relative Points

- If X-ray shows an osteoporosis bone reaction, fusion is not the ideal indication (fig. 49).
- Column (fig. 50) fusion is contraindicated for a distorted vertebra.
- Clinically, with an EMG finding of 'neurotmesis', there is no hope for a surgical result.

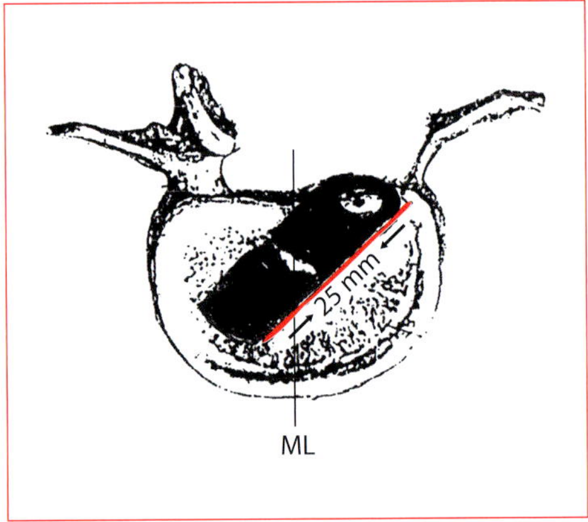

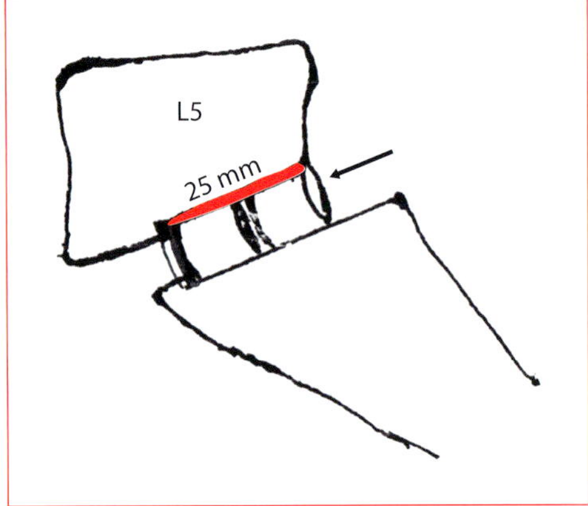

Fig. 47. Bone plugs zone needs 25 mm length for stability.

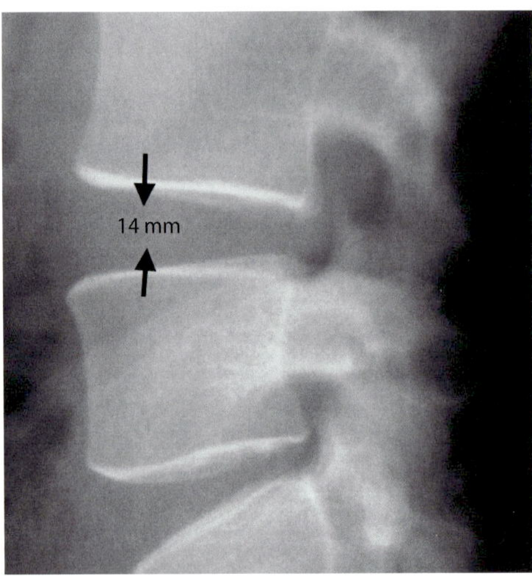

Fig. 48. 14 mm high intervertebral space represents the maximal upper limit for the insertion of 18-mm bone plugs.

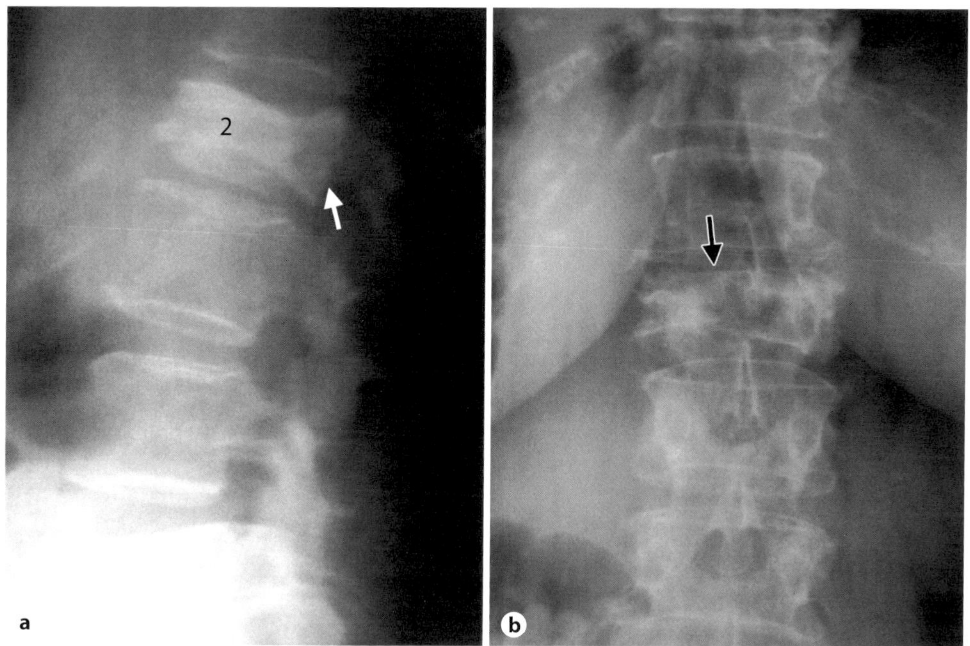

Fig. 49. a, b L2 vertebra body deformation with contraindication for bone plugs fusion.

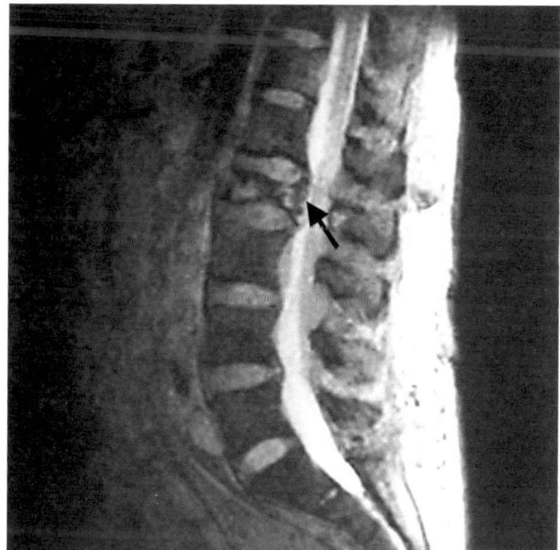

Fig. 50. MRI shows osteoporotic inflammatory deformation.

History of Oh's Temporary Marking Screw Development

The *special Oh screw* has 4 important functions during the time it stays in the body, i.e. it keeps bone plugs together for consolidation for 2 months or more.

General:

- Through 10 years of clinical development, the Oh screw has been developed through step-by-step experience since 2007.
- There are 4 morphological variations of the screws for best adaptation and stability. Easy finding and removing of the screw in the bone plugs.
- Two months following the operation, the osseous consolidation of the plugs has ended, the screw has thereby completed its task and can be removed.

Locating the Plugs by Radiological Control

The stability of the inserted plugs can be monitored by means of repeated X-rays, particularly during the initial mobilization phase of 3–14 days. The exact position of the plugs, which are relatively penetrable, cannot be determined with sufficient accuracy in most cases, especially in the lumbosacral pelvic region – the so-called body centre (see fig. 62).

Stabilization of the Plugs

For anatomical reasons, the individual plug fragment does not always have an absolutely parallel form (fig. 51). Optimum loading will be achieved if the cortical hard margins remain in the direction of forces. The screw fixes the orientation of the individual plug fragment and also prevent the bone plug from slipping back into the spinal canal (fig. 52).

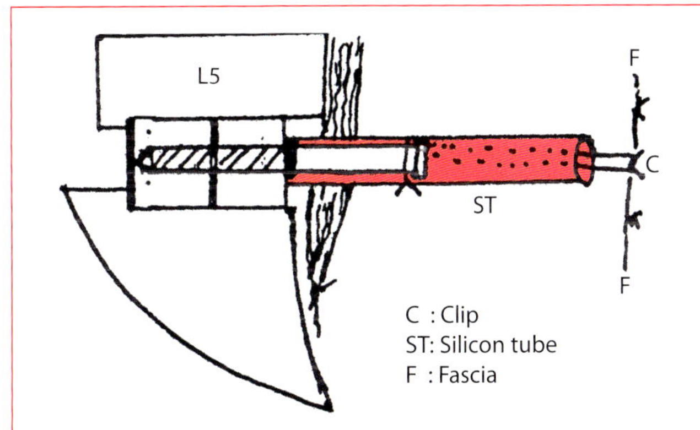

Fig. 51. Oh's temporary marking screw. ST = Silicon tube; C = clip; F = fascia.

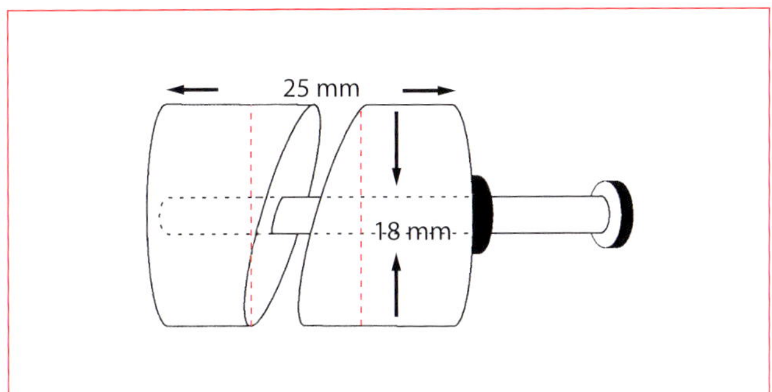

Fig. 52. Normally deformed.

Ideal Screw Position

The screw has to have exact and direct contact with the dorsal plugs (fig. 53). It is important that the ventral plug is located in a stable as possible position against the dorsal plug. If the X-ray reveals compact fixation with the screw, it means a situation of stable fusion (fig. 54).

Easy Removal of the Temporary Marking Screw

With the optimal new developed screw, it is very easy to find the head of the screw by checking with X-rays. The nerve and dura are located in the lower part of the extended head. Thanks to the silicon tube the screw can be removed without damaging dura and nerve. There are no problems with free preparation (the head of the marking screw lies in the silicon tube). The marking screw can be removed (fig. 51).

Periodic Development of Oh's Marking Screw

1st Period – Without Screw: 1990–1993

Based on clinical experience, the screw was developed step by step. The new marking screw, with its superior performance, required 10 years of design.

The first fusion operation was performed in November 1990 for instable spondylolisthesis on level L4/5 with a herniated intervertebral disc. The first 13 cases were treated without the screw. A complication developed abruptly in case 13. The patient suffered acute sciatic pain with sensomotoric weakness of nerve root L5 on the right side. There were symptoms of nerve root compression; the plugs are often not visible at X-ray in a sitting person if the patient has a thick pelvis. An emergency operation was performed; the dorsal plug luxated particularly into the spine canal. Nerve root L5 was compressed (table 2, patient 13).

After this event, in the following operations the author regularly used a screw to fix the inserted plugs together (fig. 53a, b). Regular X-rays were done to check the position of the screw.

Case: 1st Patient with Oh's Fusion

46-year-old male (no screw).

Diagnosis: Sciatic pain on both sides with IVHD with instable spondylolisthesis L5/S1 (fig. 54–57).

Therapy: Removal of the herniated disc and fusion with bone plugs.

Operation: 06.11.1990.

Control: 9 years later the author invited the patient for a checkup. The patient was in a good condition, having no back pain or pain in the legs. X-ray showed good consolidation (fig. 54).

2nd Period – Normal Screw Application: 1993–1997

With the ventral plug seats stable, it can happen that the dorsal plug could slip into the spinal canal (table 2). To avoid slippage of the dorsal plug, both the ventral and dorsal plugs were fixed together with a normal screw (fig. 53). To check the stability of the screw and the plugs regular X-rays were done.

With obese patients, the pelvic region is not easy to check visually, but thanks to the screw checking is now easier (fig. 55).

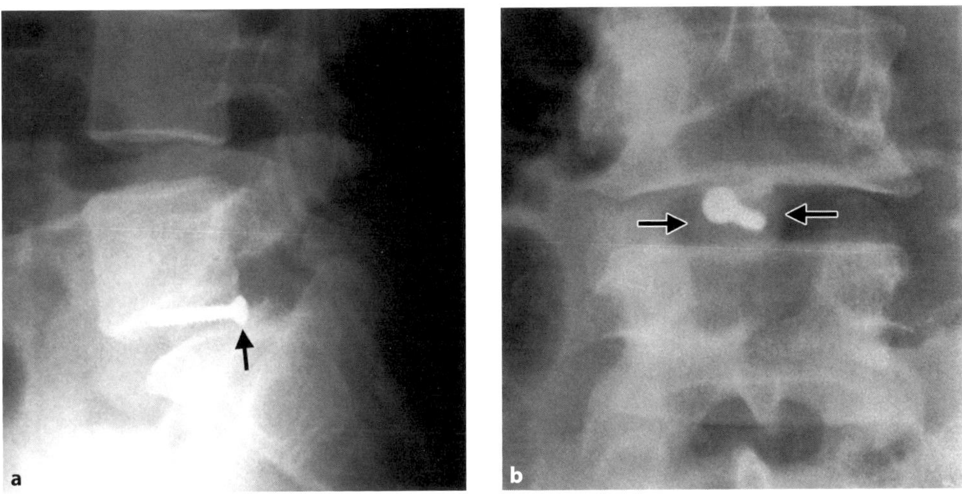

Fig. 53. a Marking screw visible only. Dorsal plug not visible. Ventral plug not visible. Normal screw fixation. **b** Optimal screw and plug position.

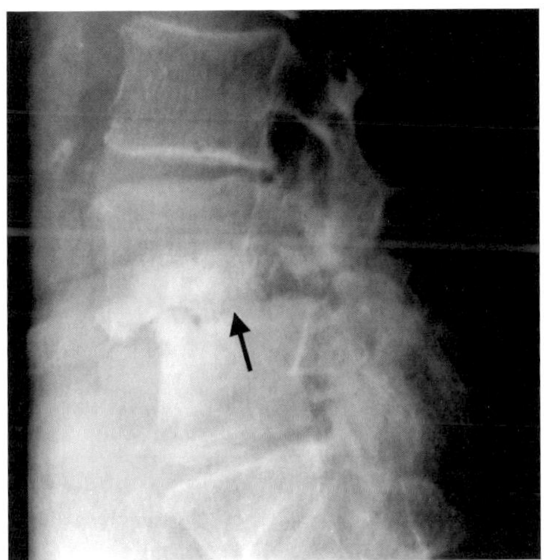

Fig. 54. Fusion operation performed under theoretical consideration without screw. First attempt with excellent results.

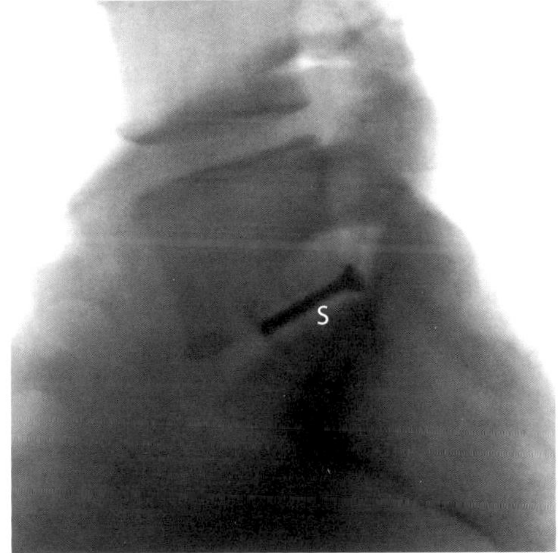

Fig. 55. With pelvic shadow no clear visibility of fusion plugs. Good visibility of fixed marking screw.

Table 2. Periodic development

	Period					
	1990–1993	1993	1993–1997	1997–1998	1999–2000	from 2000
Temporal						
Marking screw	not used until patient 13	patient 13 dorsal plug luxation into canal (complication)	normal screw	1st Oh's designed screw (too long shaft partly protruding)	2nd Oh's screw (1/2 screw and 1/2 shaft part)	3rd Oh's screw no adhesion (easy to remove)
	fig. 52	fig. 53	fig. 54	fig. 55a, b	fig. 56	fig. 57

3rd Period – Extended Head Screw: 1997–1998

Oh's long-head screw was designed in 1997 (fig. 56a, b).

As already stated, some weeks after the fusion operation the screw has to be taken out. The reason for the further development of the screw was because from time to time the author had difficulties in finding the screw in order to remove it. It is a delicate procedure, protecting the nerve root and dura which were stuck to the screw. It could happen that after removal of the screw, the patient would again complain of radiating pain.

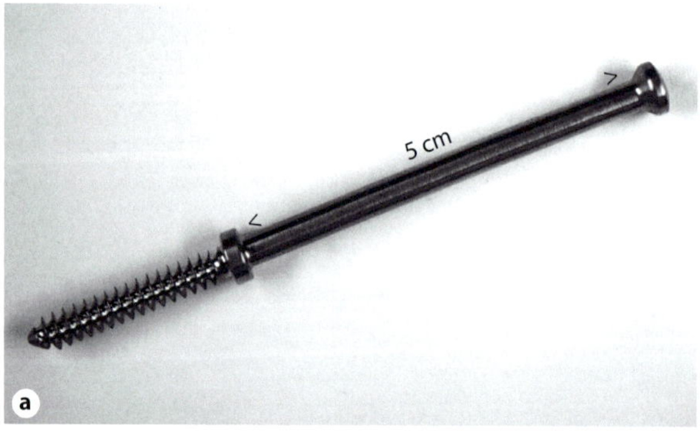

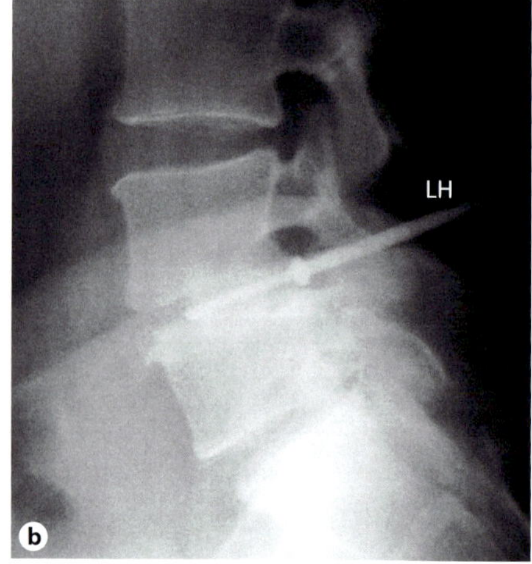

Fig. 56. a, b Temporarily used long head (LH) screw.

This was a reason to think about finding a new model of screw, and in 1997 this new model was designed. This screw had an extending head (fig. 56). The advantage of this screw was that it was easy to find for removal, because the head of the screw was lying under the muscle. The disadvantage was because of the long head of the screw, it compressed superficial muscle and produced muscle pain.

4th Period – Shortened Head Part: 1999–2000

The long-head screw was used for 1 year and was inserted in several patients. Most of the patients complained about back muscle pain. The reason for this was the 50 mm long head of the screw, which was located under the fascia layer. From 1999, the long screw was shortened to 25 mm (fig. 57a), now the head of the screw is located in a deep muscle layer (fig. 57b). *Result:* The patients no longer complain about back pain.

By removing the screw from the junction, the screw head shows dura and nerve root adhesion; a silicon tube covering the head of screw prevents adhesion.

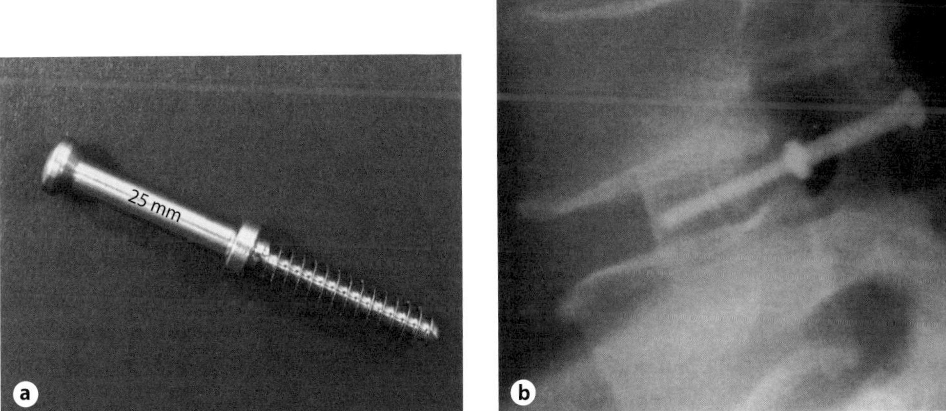

Fig. 57. a, b Optimal fixing-marking of plugs screw.

There are three different lengths of the screw threads (fig. 57c). The length depends on the size of the plugs and represents between 20, 22 and 24 mm (fig. 57d).

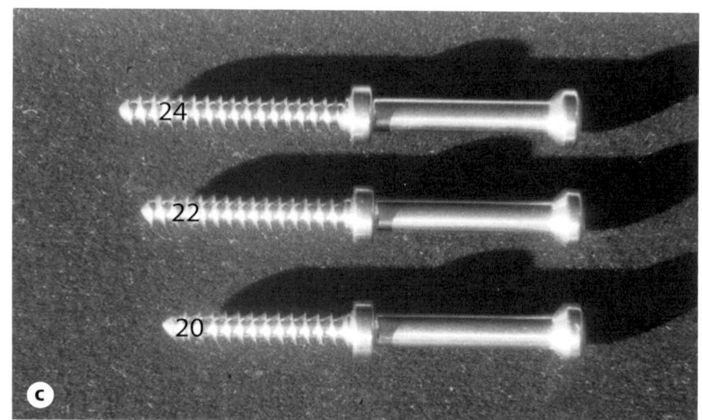

Fig. 57. c Different screw lengths.

5th Period: From 2000

Oh's Temporary Marking Screw
It emerged that the additional part of the screw needed a preventative measure against adhesion with dura and nerve root. Since the last additional screw model has been in use, there are no longer any problems in removing the screws.

Results: Patients have no further complaints.

Additional Parts
- Silicon covers (extended head)
- Marking clips (marking silk end subcutaneous ligament)

A silicon tube covers the extended head of the screw, helping to prevent nerve root and dura matter adhesion.

The extended screw head is connected with a black silk thread, which is easily visible in the context of an operation (fig. 58a). The end of the silk thread is fixed subcutaneously with the fascia and marked with a silver clip (fig. 58b) and it is easy to find.

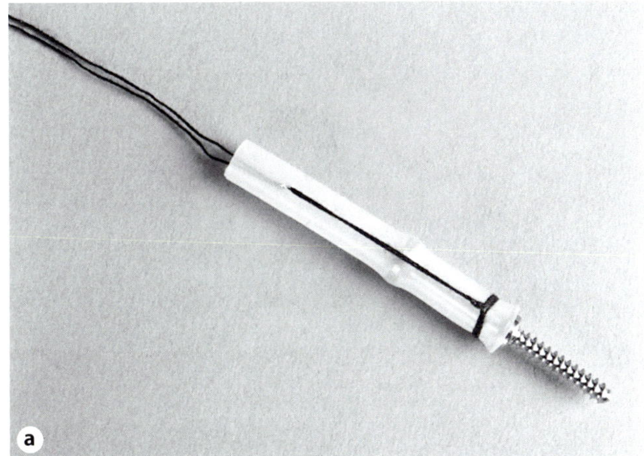

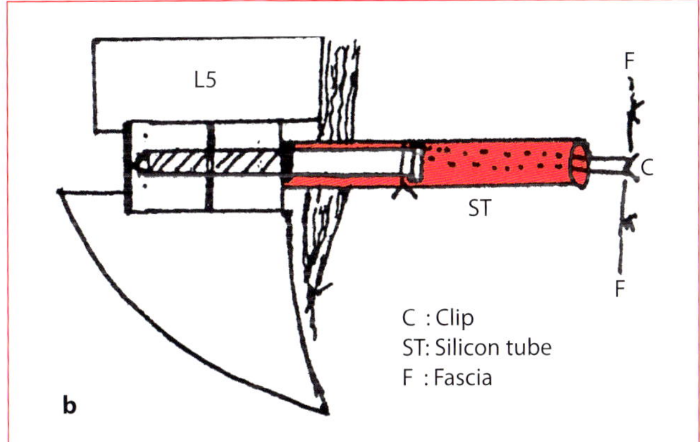

Fig. 58. a, b Oh's temporary marking bone plugs screw.

Aspects of Autologous Bone Plugs

Where Plugs Are Taken From

Figure 59 illustrates removed ventral edge ileac bone. Usually, the diameter of the ileac bone plugs measures 10–14 mm. It is necessary to use two pieces of plugs (fixed together these have an ideal length between 20 and 25 mm; fig. 51). The edge of the ileac bone consists of hard bone to maximize collapse protection (fig. 60a, b).

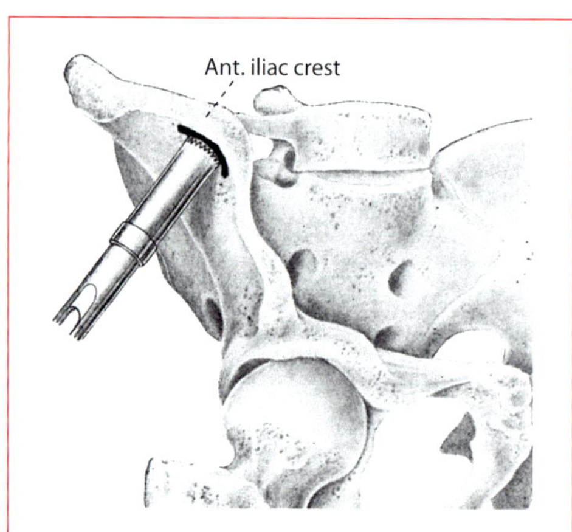

Fig. 59. Plug cutter is placed below the crest of the ileum to obtain as long a plug as possible with cortical bone plate on both ends.

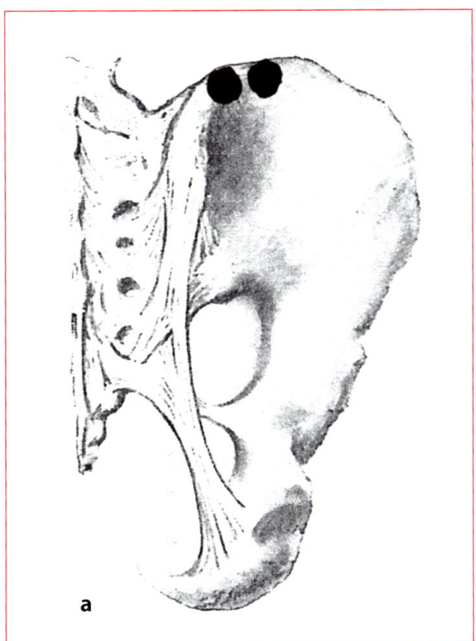

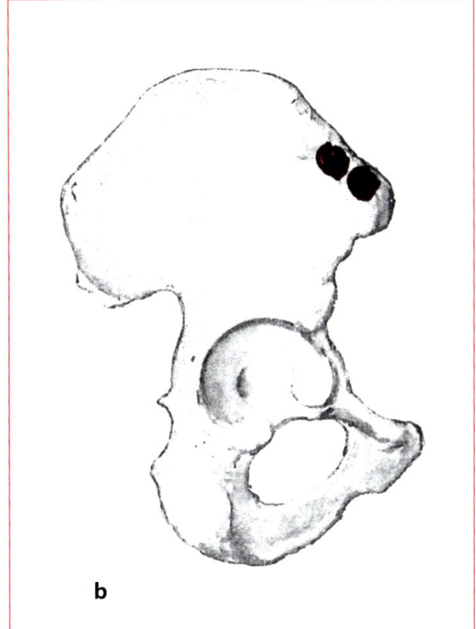

Fig. 60. Plug cut area. **a** Inside ileum. **b** Outside ileum.

Bone Plug Aspects

The two ossified plugs – which are now fixed together as one living cylindrical plug – show 4 characteristic aspects:

- Living plug function
- Small, jewel shaped
- Architectonic aspects
- Efficient activity

Living Plug

At radiological examination, the strong osteosclerotic shadow of the united plug has to confirm its living situation (fig. 61a, b). No non-union!

The research work for the plug was performed radiologically. The plain X-ray shows the plug (operation was 5 years ago, 1993; fig. 61a) compared to the same view 18 years later, 2008 (fig. 61b) – the dorsal plug is hardly visible. Significant CT checking clearly shows a living plug (fig. 62a, b).

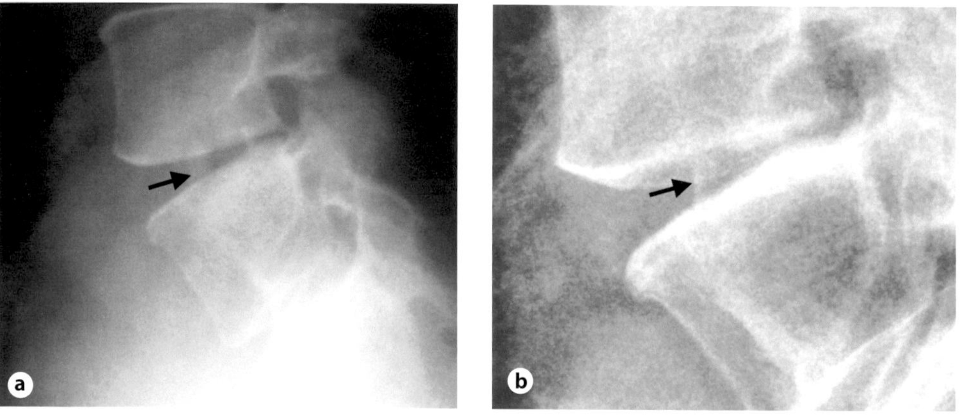

Fig. 61. a, b Similar consolidation with plug and column is seen when comparing operation of 1993 and X-ray control of 2008 (15 years later).

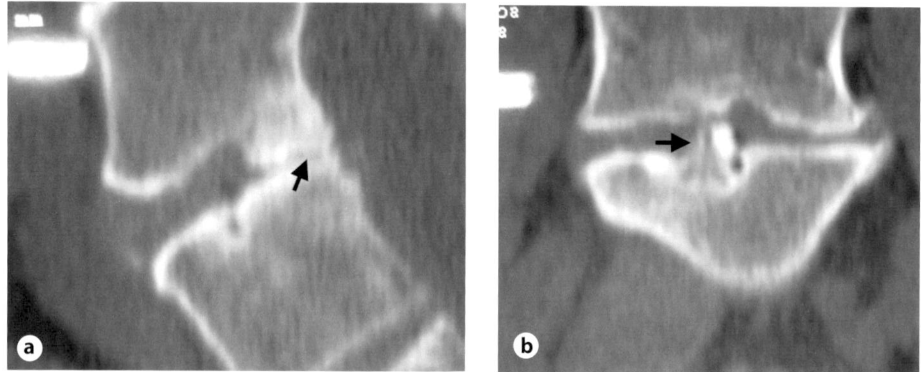

Fig. 62. a, b 15 years later: plug control – perfect ossification.

Small Cylindrical Bone Plug

Two plugs are now ossified into one plug with a cylindrical contour (fig. 63). According to the measurements of the plugs, the carrying capacity is approximately 5–6 cm^3 (fig. 62). This living small plug is located in the central body region (fig. 64).

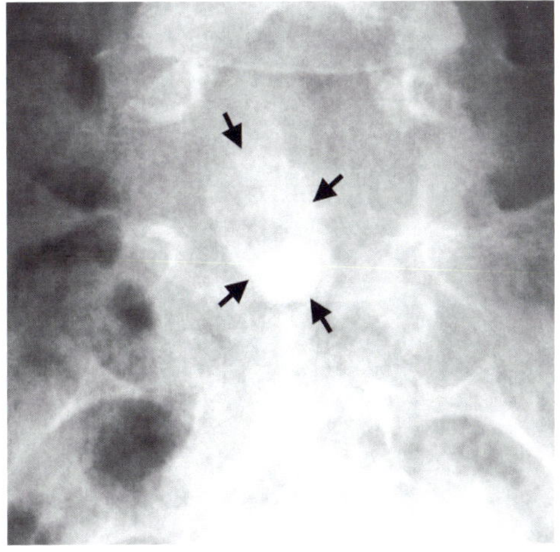

Fig. 63. Jewel-like united plug.

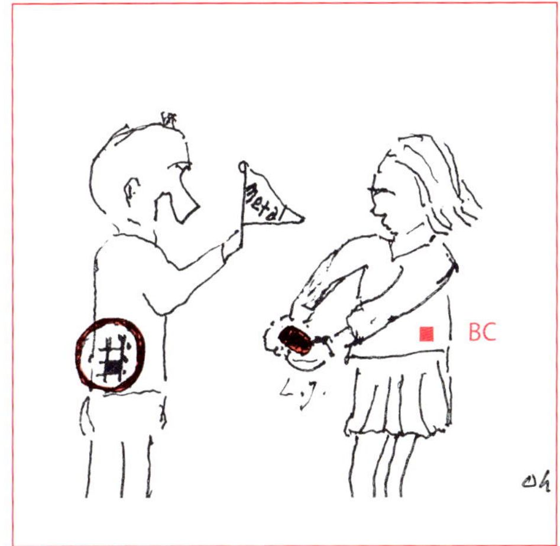

Fig. 64. Living jewel.

Architectonic Aspects

Carrying capacity

For example:

The length of the plug is 20–25 mm and 14–16 mm wide

$8^2 \cdot \pi \cdot l$

Radius 16 mm (50% = 8 mm)

$8 \times 8 = 64$

64×3.14 (pi) = 200.96

200.96×25 (length) = 5,024 mm^3 (5.024 cm^3)

This carrying capacity covers the loading of the upper part of the human body.

Body Center (BC)

The body center combines carrying and neurological functions (fig. 65).

The carrying function of the body center is more important. Neuroanatomic function structures are located here. The following dysfunctions in the body center can occur:

- Walking disturbance (neuro-orthopedic)
- Bladder dysfunction and stool disturbance
- Sexual disturbances
- The part of the body center which functions by coordinating carrying and neurological activity (fig. 65)

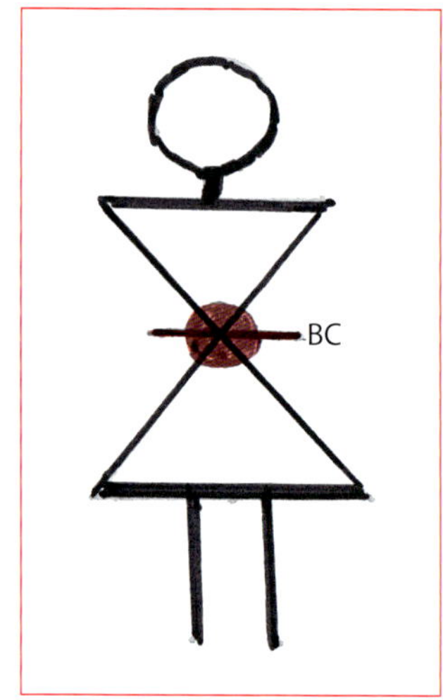

Fig. 65. Neuro-orthopedic coordination center. BC = Body center.

Efficient Activity

Bone plugs consist of two different histological structures: soft on the inside, with a hard bony plate on the outside (fig. 66).

MRI/CT shows an impressive picture of the living plug of cortical hard margin (fig. 67a, b).

This effective part avoids collapse of the intervertebral space. It has an important function and is additionally spread 4 mm with a spreader.

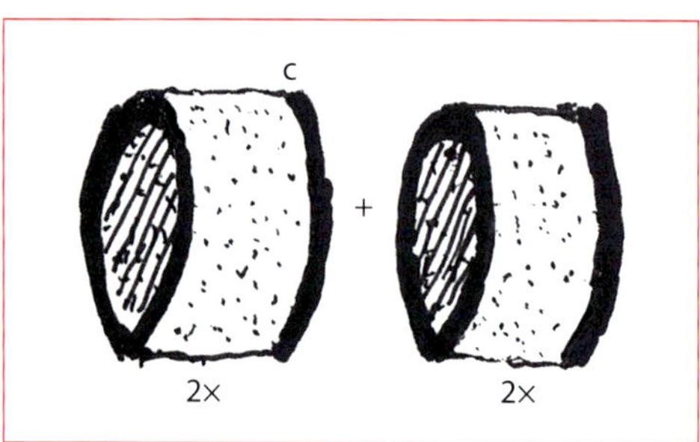

Fig. 66. Cortical plug hard plate protects for compact fusion. C = Cortical plate.

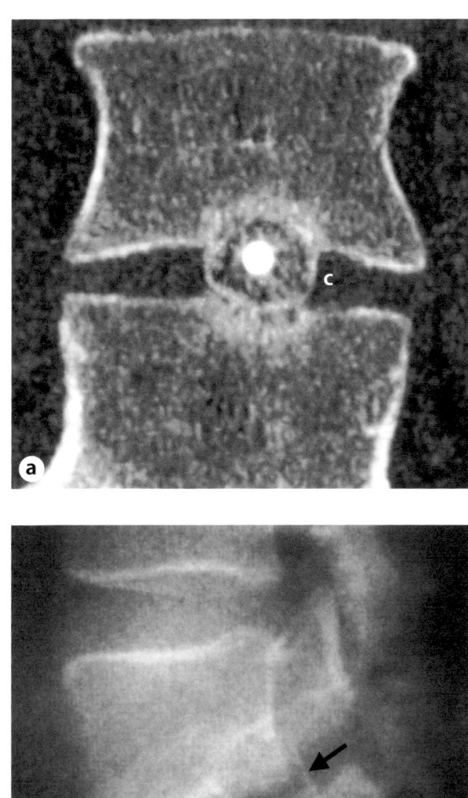

Fig. 67. a, b Hard cortical plates are clearly seen.

Operative Technical Procedure

Based on many years of experience in cervical bone plugs fusion-operations, the author developed bone plugs fusion in the lumbar spine using autologous bone for diverse instabilities (fig. 68).

The UOPIF (unilateral oblique posterior intervertebral fusion) as well as deep anatomical, physiological and radiological knowledge are prerequisites for a good operative technique without the use of foreign substances. The operative technique respects topographical situations without taking foreign substances into consideration.

To achieve a satisfactory surgical result, the following are critical points to be taken into consideration:

(1) Target line for fusion
(2) Unilateral extended laminectomy
(3) Special instruments
(4) Drilling procedure
(5) Size of drill, hole and bone plugs
(6) Compact plugs fusion
(7) Oh's temporary *marking screw* fixation
(8) Removing Oh's screw

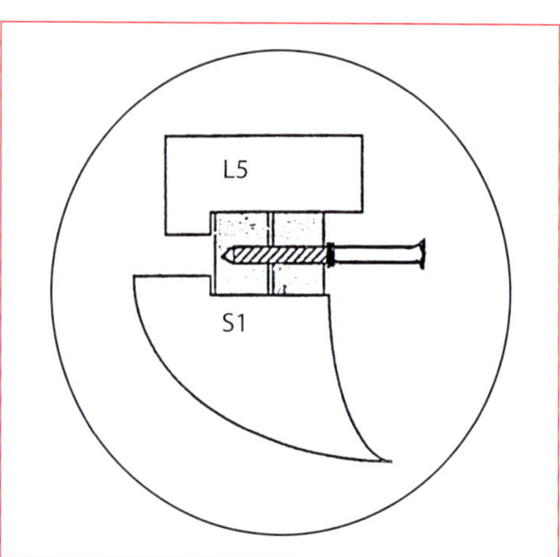

Fig. 68. Standard bone plugs fusion (UOPIF).

UOPIF

• Unilateral	(U)	UO
• Oblique	(O)	
• Posterior	(P)	PI
• Interbody	(I)	
• Fusions	(F)	F

UOPIF thus means perfect osseous consolidation with surgically transplanted bone plugs procedure (fig. 70).

The result is a blocked L4/5 vertebra without foreign bodies (fig. 70).

Target Line for Bone Plugs Fusion

- Anatomical views show vertebral column of adults with average 3 cm ventrodorsal length, 4 cm long lateral view (fig. 69).
- Ventrodorsal is displaced by 10 mm and therefore measures 30 mm interbody space. A long isolation of the facet joint of the wrists generating necrotic porotic alternation and cystic contents is rare.
- To do the fusion, it is necessary to have a space of at least 25 mm diameter for the enlarged hemilaminectomy (fig. 71).
- Two bone plugs are normally required – together these have a length of about 25 mm. Approximately 5 mm wall for the ventral region for the stabilisation of the ventral plugs.
- The edge at the rear of the dorsal plug should form a line with the upper vertebra.

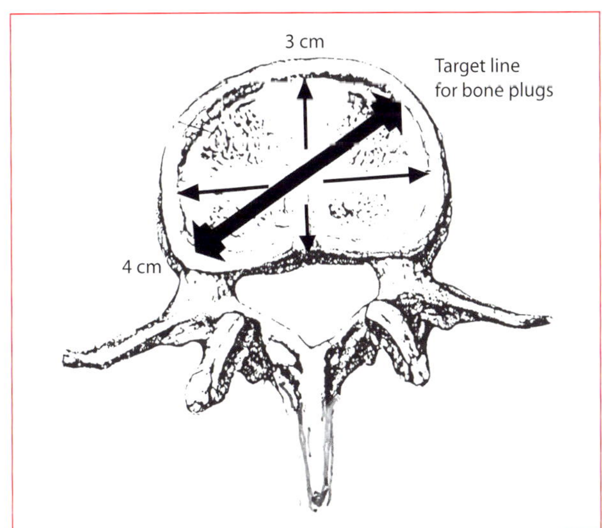

Fig. 69. Ideal line for drilling – unilateral oblique posterior.

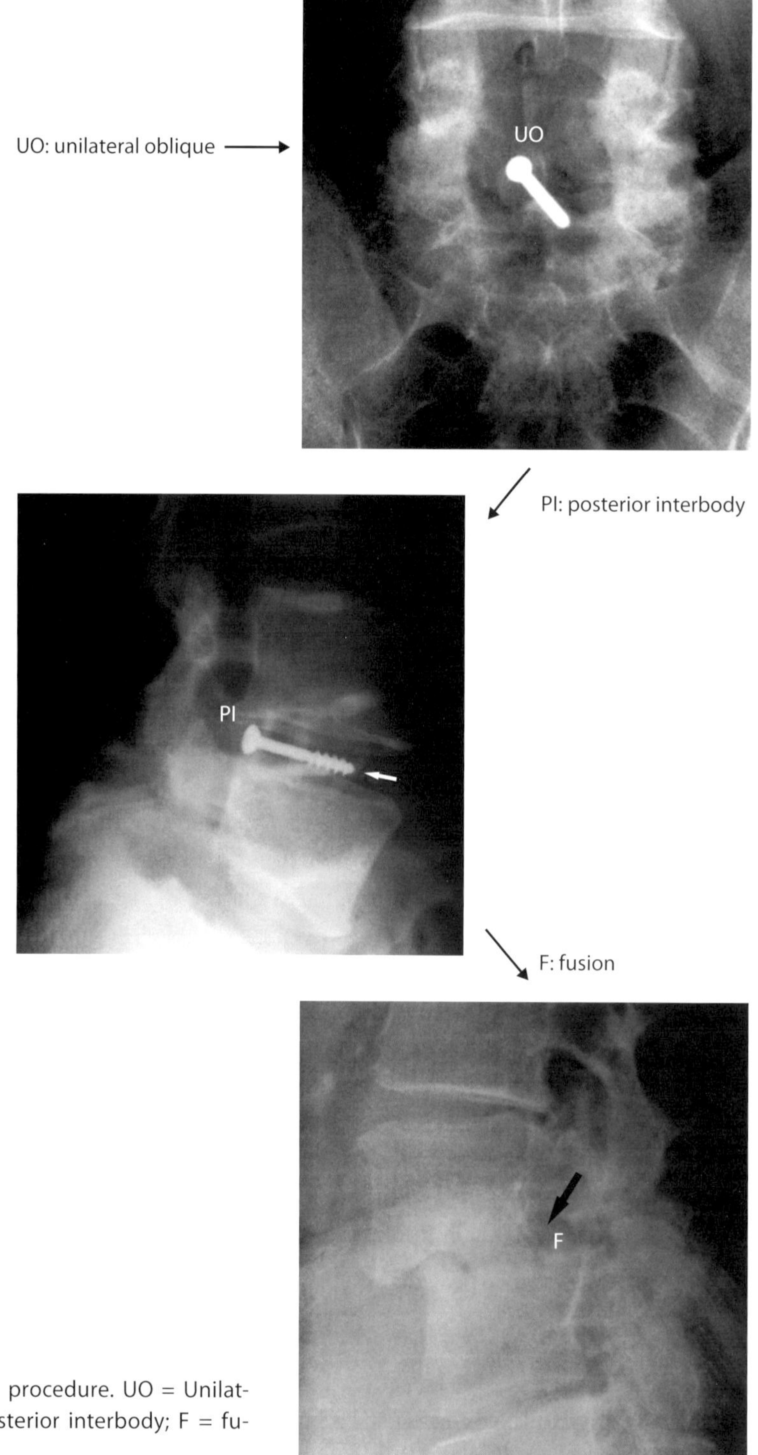

Fig. 70. UOPIF fusion procedure. UO = Unilateral oblique; PI = posterior interbody; F = fusion.

Extended One-Sided Laminectomy

Based on conventional techniques, the first part of the operation involves removing the spinal arch, exposing and removing a herniated intervertebral disc, if present, and osseous relief of stenotic reactions. For the insertion of plugs, it is necessary to perform an enlarged laminectomy (fig. 71).

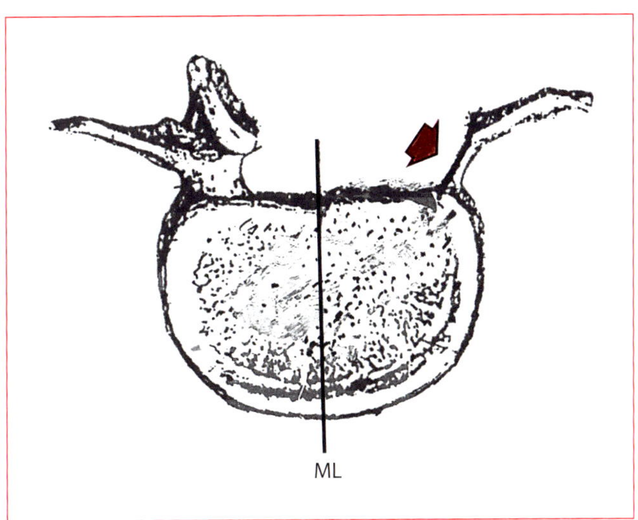

Fig. 71. Extended one-sided laminectomy.

Special Instruments

For this technique some special instruments are required (fig. 72–74):

- Nerve root hook
- Spreader

At the end of the nerve root hook there is a tooth, which helps to protect against slipping (fig. 72).

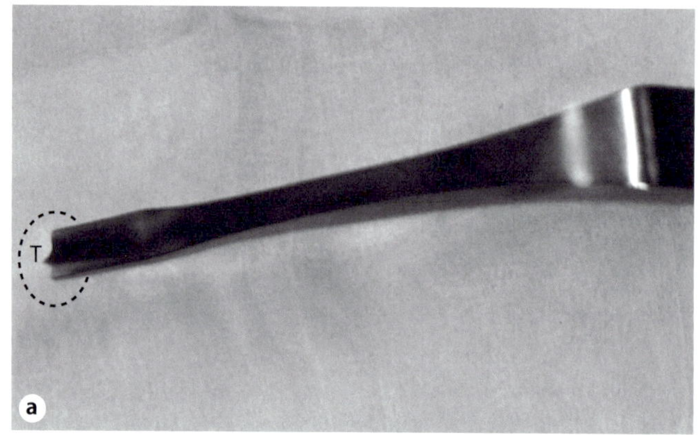

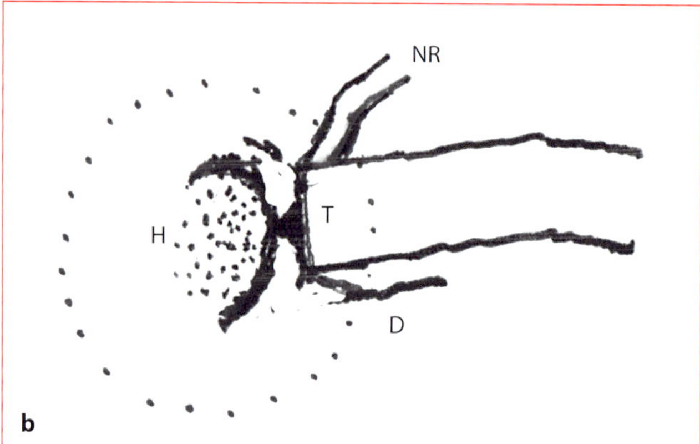

Fig. 72. a, b Hook of nerve root special. T = Tooth; H = hole; D = dura; NR = nerve root.

Drilling:

(a) Nerve roots hooks (fig. 72) for drilling process.

(b) Stable fixation of spreader in opposite intervertebral space and X-ray control (fig. 73).

(c) After making space for drilling, the intervertebral space has to be checked by X-ray.

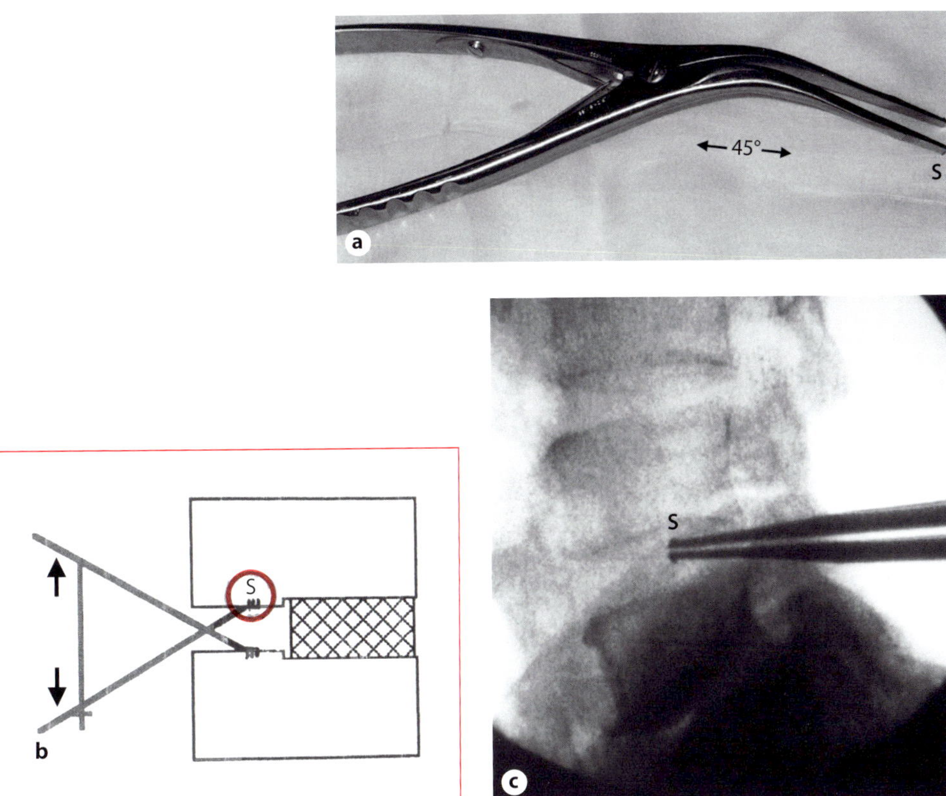

Fig. 73. a, b Spreader interspace special. S = Spike. **c** X-ray control spreader in the sitting position. The spreader has small spikes on its end (fig. 74) preventing it from slipping.

Drilling – Procedure

Middle position drill with removal of cortical plate on both sides. Drilling is checked with X-ray (fig. 74), and removal of both sides of the hard plate is achieved (fig. 73b).

The bone drill is applied from one side unilaterally, drilling oblique towards the opposite (fig. 75a) and crossing the midline of the vertebral body (fig. 75b). Drill removing the thin hard plate in the intervertebral room is completed in order to allow rapid vertebral column and plugs consolidation.

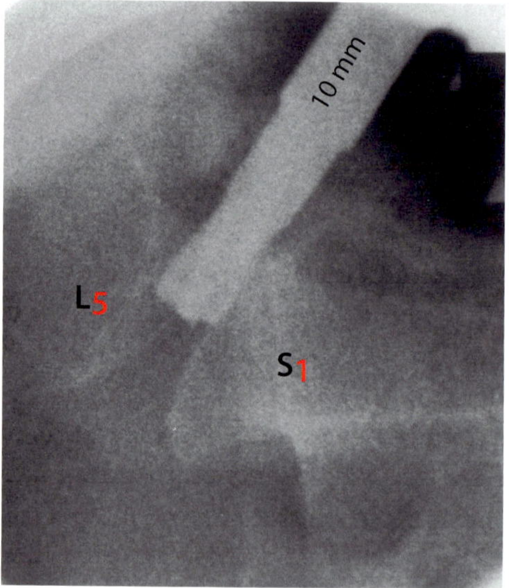

Fig. 74. 8 mm interbody space – drill 10 mm.

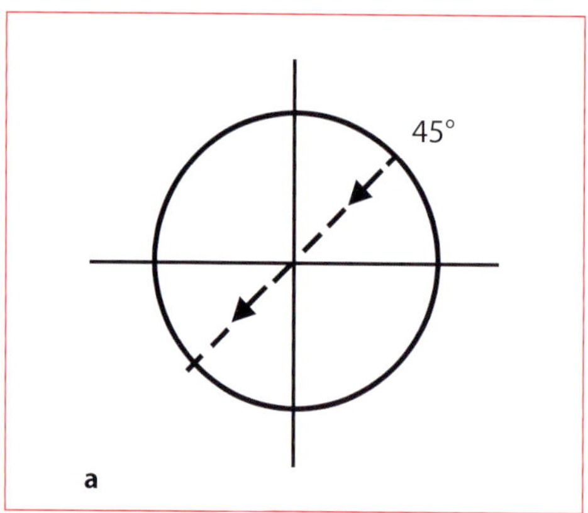

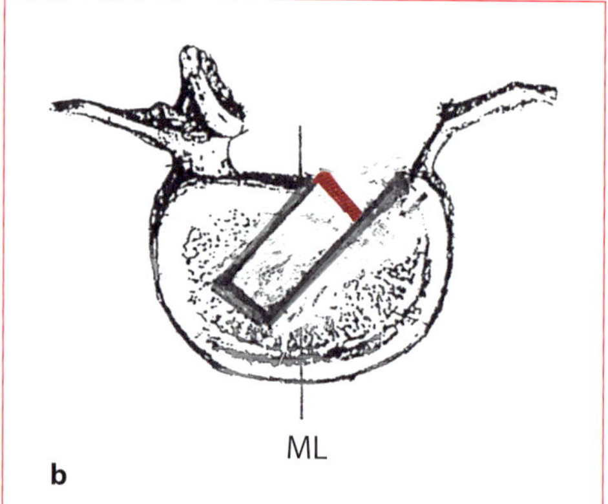

Fig. 75. a, b Unilateral oblique (45°) position for drilling.

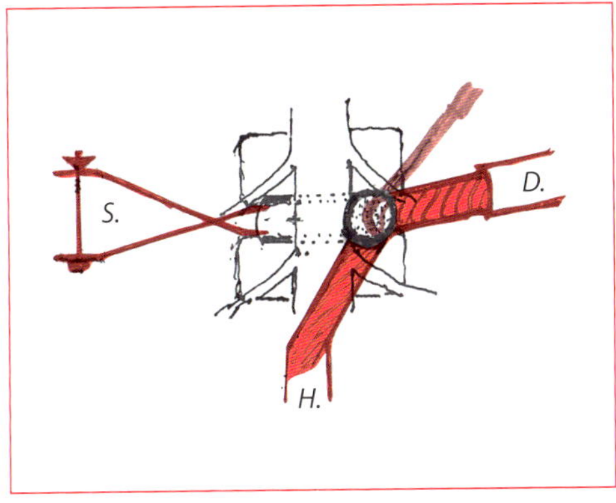

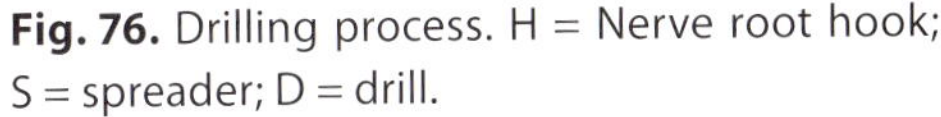
Fig. 76. Drilling process. H = Nerve root hook; S = spreader; D = drill.

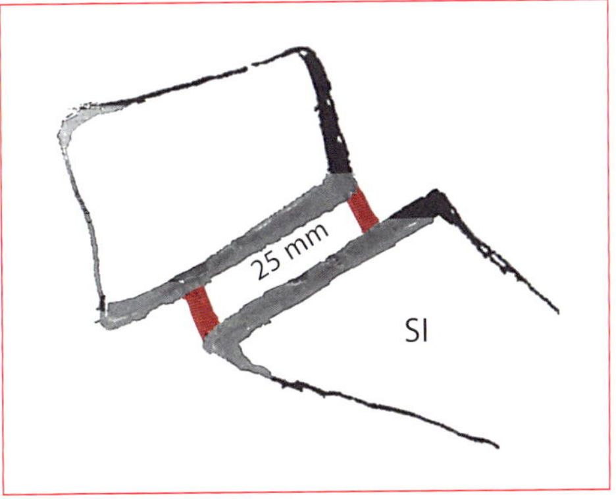

Fig. 77. Lateral view: 20–25 mm length – ideal for plugs insertion.

Prior to preparation for drilling without damage to the nerve root or dura, the following key points are important in the fusion procedure:

- 2 assistants are required to protect 2 nerve roots
- 2 suctions for blood suction (in case of strong bleeding)

One assistant must hold the nerve root hook (fig. 76) and the other assistant holds one of the suctions. In case of strong bleeding, two suctions are required during the drilling. In this end phase of the fusion operation, it is absolutely essential to have sufficient personnel for manual help. The technique of the operation shows the importance of the first phase of the drilling procedure (fig. 77) and insertion of the plugs.

For protecting nerve roots, a special hook is required (fig. 72).

For the intervertebral space, special instruments (spreader) are required, which the author constructed himself (fig. 72, 74).

Size of Drill Hole and Bone Plug

Compared to the cervical spine, for example, considerably greater loads occur in interbody bone plugs transplantation in the lumbar spine. In order to take up these forces, stable interbody support is absolutely essential. If the remaining intervertebral space measures 10 mm, then we initially drill to 12 mm and the spread to 16 mm (table 3). Anatomical topographical mobility and loading function compared very different aspects. For ideal fusions bigger lumbar are better than cervical plugs (table 3).

Lower or higher starting values are correspondingly taken into account. The surfaces of the upper plate and lower plate are trimmed in order to ensure good osseous incorporation of the plugs.

Important Factors

Compared to cervical fusion, lumbar fusion is technically more demanding for the surgeon, because of the anatomical features (nerve roots and dura).

Inserting a plug with a diameter 4 mm bigger than the hole must be done carefully and with precision (fig. 78).

Table 3. Compare plugs insertion by stability

Region	IVBS	Bohring	Plugs
Cervical	8 mm	10 mm	12 mm
Lumbar	8 mm	10 mm	14 mm
Interbody space	**Hole**	**Plugs (2 ×)**	**Fusion length**
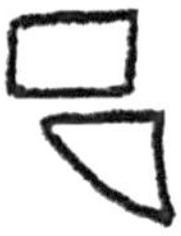	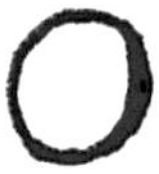	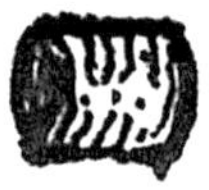	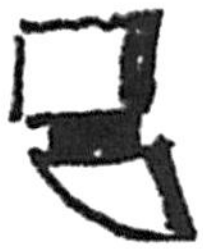
6 mm	8 mm	12 mm	20–25 mm
8 mm	10 mm	14 mm	20–25 mm
10 mm	12 mm	16 mm	20–25 mm
12 mm	14 mm	18 mm	20–25 mm

Bone plugs
Size = 10–18 mm diameter (no more than 18 mm).
Length = 20–25 mm.
Plugs = 2 pieces (approximately 12 mm + 12 mm).
Temporary = fixation of the plugs with Oh's marking screw.

Compact Fitting with Several Bone Plugs

- Single layer fusion

A bone drill is applied from one side, drilling obliquely towards the opposite side to cross the midline of the vertebral body (fig. 79).

To take into account the considerably greater axial interbody lead compared to the cervical spine, two or three bi-cortical bone fragments form the iliac crest which are formed together into an actual bone plug are used.

For example for a stable fusion:

- 10 mm interbody space (fig. 80a and c)
- 12 mm drilling hole (fig. 81a)
- 16 mm bone plugs are inserted into the 12-mm drilled interbody space (fig. 80b)
- Unilateral oblique fusion (fig. 81a, b)
- Plugs fixed with screw (fig. 82)

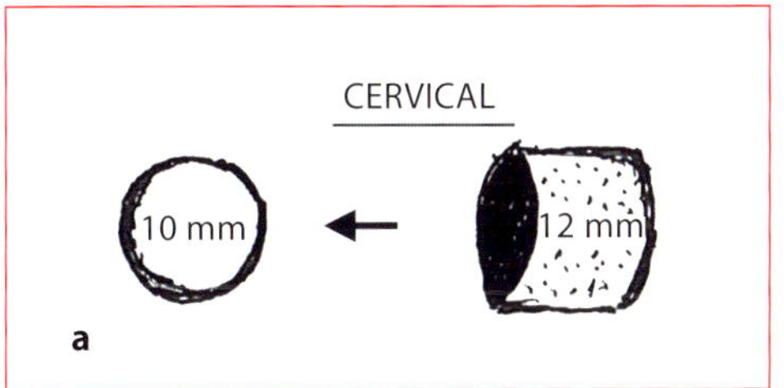

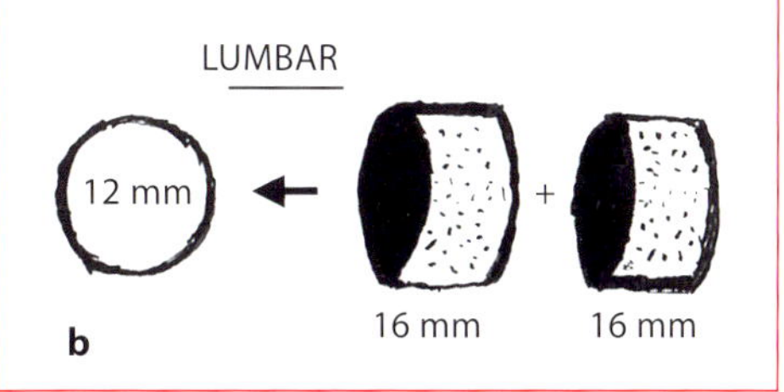

Fig. 78. a, b Relation hole: between plug in the cervical and lumbar column.

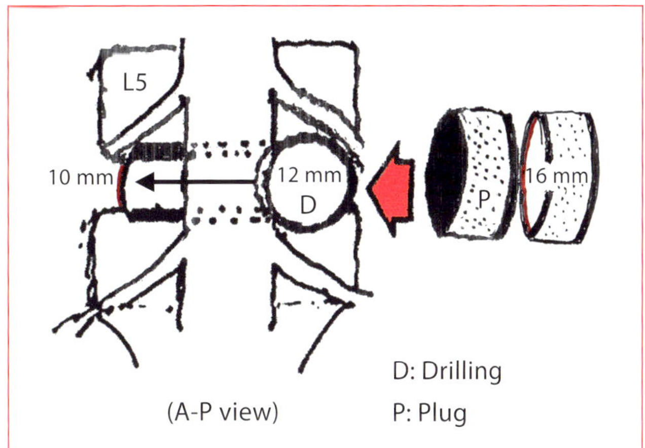

Fig. 79. Stable fusion.

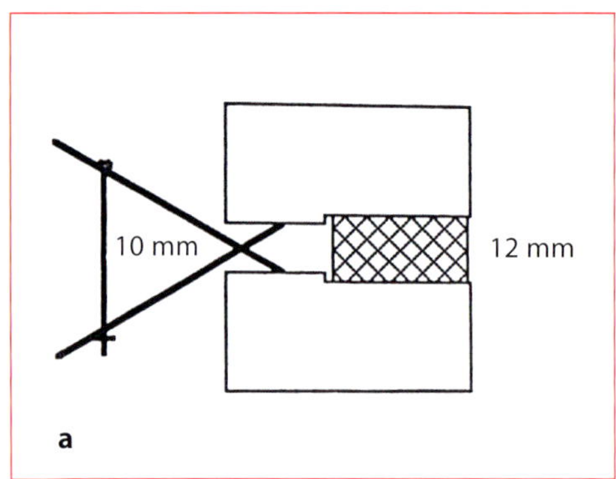

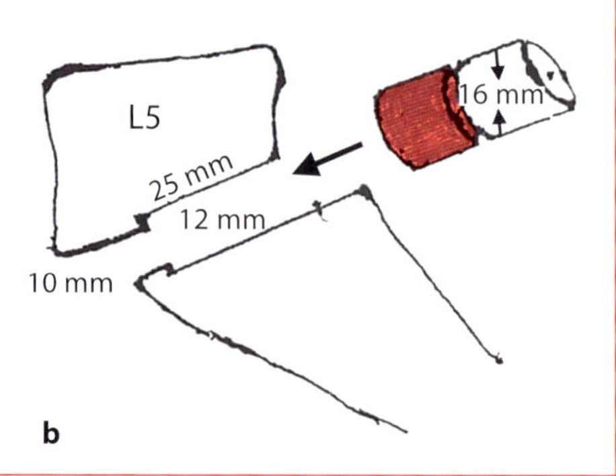

Fig. 80. a, b Interbody space 10 mm. Drilled space 12 mm. 2 plugs fitting 16 mm.

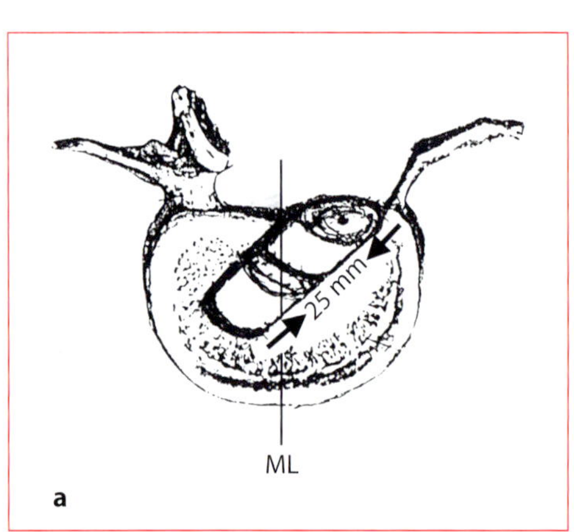

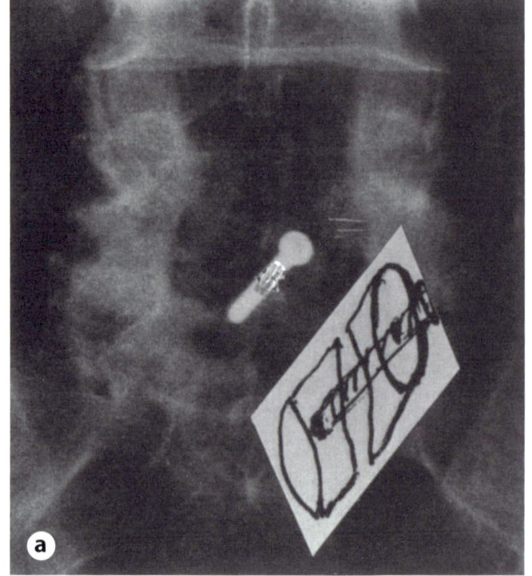

Fig. 81. a, b A-P view: unilateral oblique fusion.

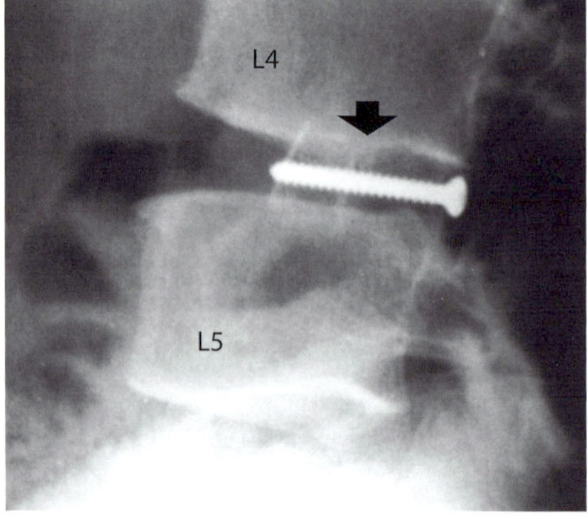

Fig. 82. Lateral view: posterior intervertebral fusion.

Double-Layer Fusion

Five cases of applying double-layer fusion by double-layer spondylolisthesis were performed.

Double segmental ventral displacement: L4/5 and L5/S1 (fig. 83). Clinically, the patients mostly suffered constant back and radiating pains in the lower extremities. These were frequently accompanied by neurological deficits.

There are three types of different causes, such as ventral and dorsal, stair-like displaced (fig. 42).

Bone plugs fusion was performed on ventrally displaced vertebrae with the cross-oblique approach (fig. 84–88).

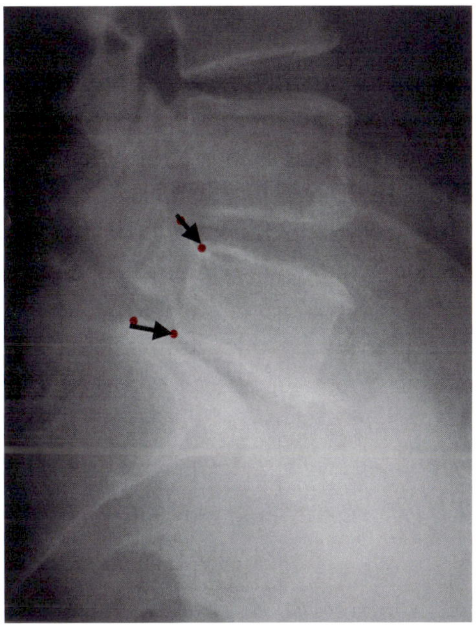

Fig. 83. Double-layer 'ventral type' spondylolisthesis: L4/5 and L5/S1.

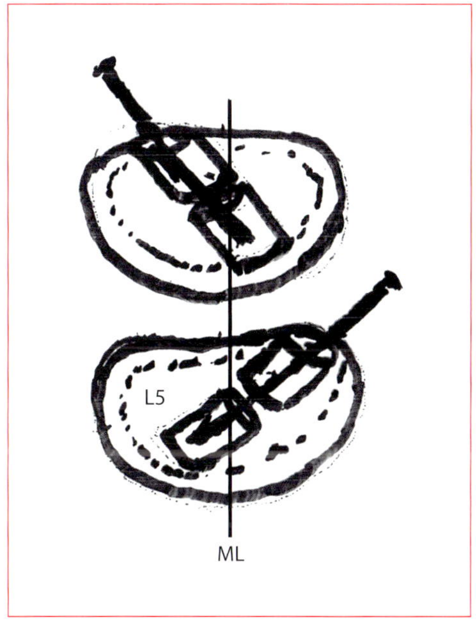

Fig. 84. For stable equilibrium, plugs are maintained in crossing oblique fusion.

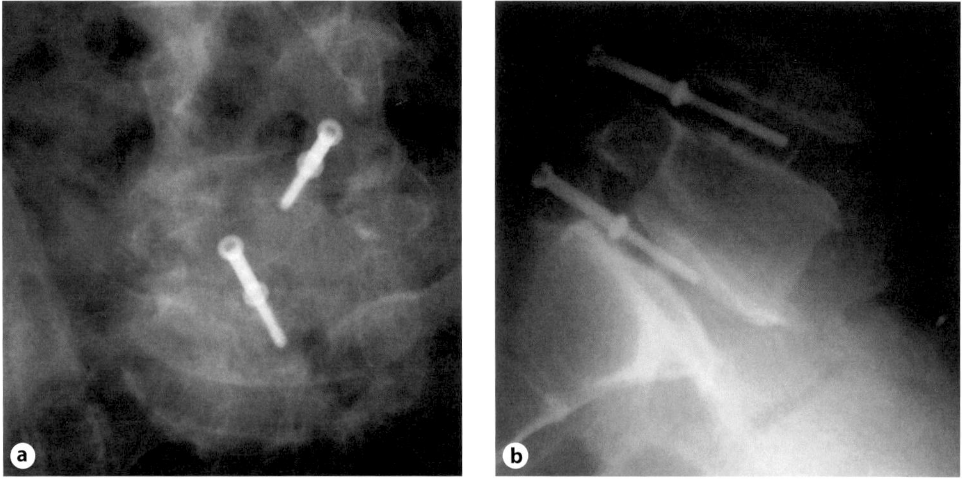

Fig. 85. a, b Double-layer spondylolisthesis L5/S1 + L4/5. Diverse crossing fusion performed.

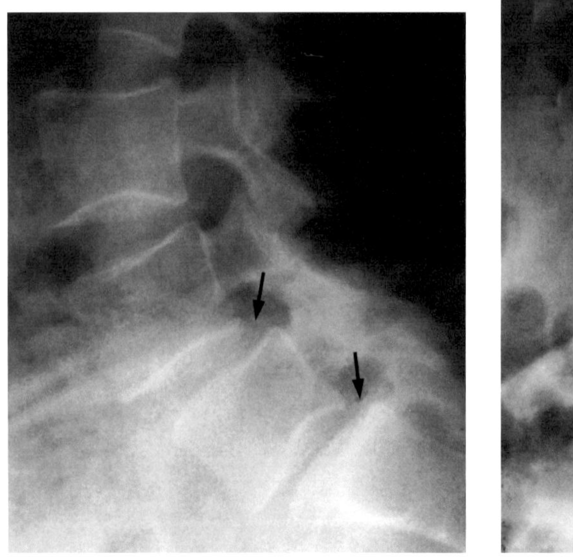

Fig. 86. Double stair-like displacement L4/5 and L5/S1.

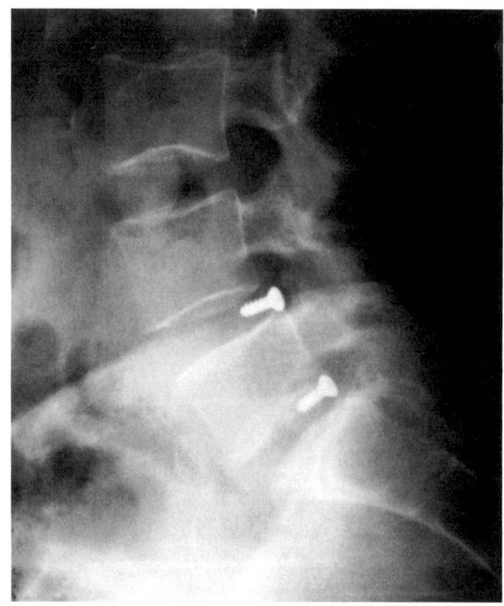

Fig. 87. Marking screw for plug control.

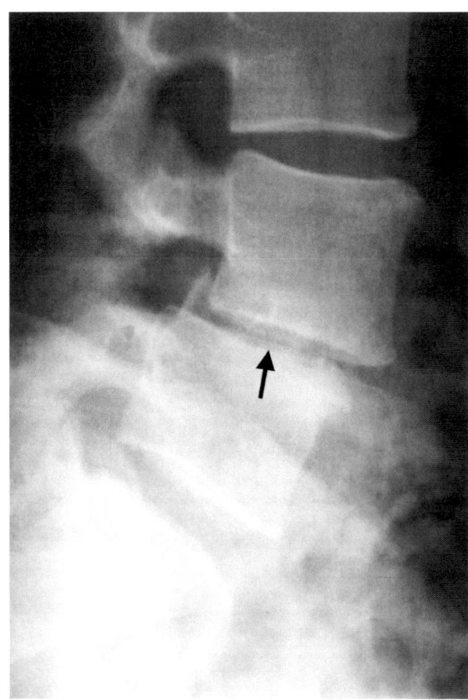

Fig. 88. L4/5 fusion results in homogeneous compact ossification, as in congenital 'block' vertebra column.

Comments

The double segment plug fusion operative technique has been performed on fewer cases, and is not as simple to do (fig. 85–88).

UOPIF fusion is looking to maintain 360° load balance and co-ordination of the left facets against the right facets; achievement of alternative fitting is important (fig. 84, 85). The author had operated on a few patients where he did not remove the screw. The reason for this was because some patients were very heavy or quite old. In these cases, an agreement with the patients to this effect was always in place before the operation. If somebody wished to keep the screw, a smaller special screw was used (fig. 87).

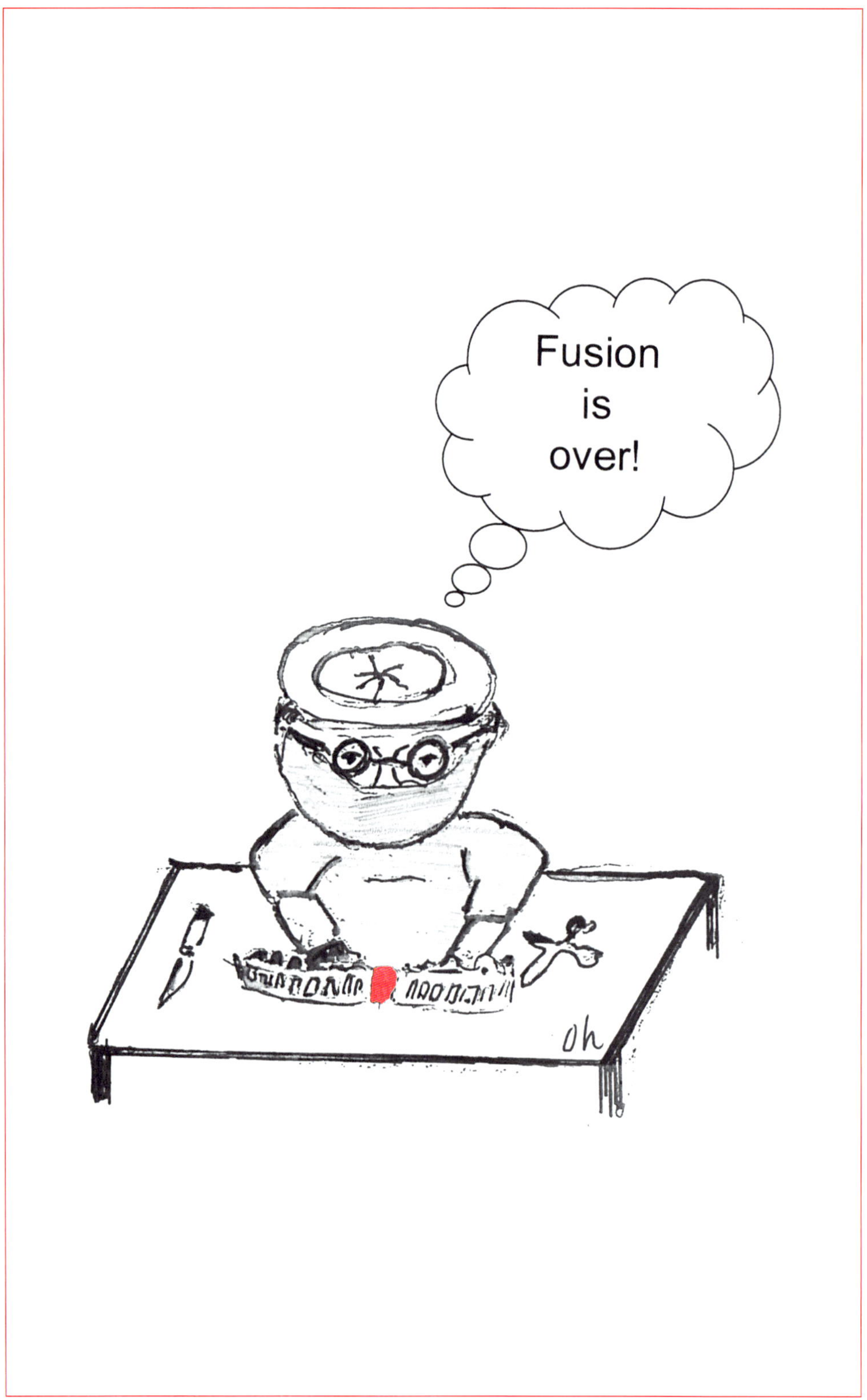
Fusion
is
over!
oh

Routine Postoperative Checks (Plug and Screw)

Routine plugs checks:

- Mobilization of the patients within 24 h
- X-ray check of the plugs after:

    24 h (operating room)

    3 days postoperatively

    2 weeks postoperatively

    1 month postoperatively

About 1 month later, if the plugs are still in a stable position, no more X-rays check-ups are indicated.

Plug Shadows

Four kinds of different plug shadows are given:

Both plugs are not visible (fig. 89a)

X-ray shows both plugs (fig. 89b)

Ventral plug visible (fig. 89c)

Only dorsal plug is visible (fig. 89d)

Normally plugs are not visible or not easily visible with plain X-ray. Therefore for checking on the plugs, it is important that the Oh's screw be located at the precisely correct point, which means also an ideal position for the plugs (fig. 89a–d).

For the author, the reason for this is not clear.

Some doctors reckon this is because the surgeons' work has not been done correctly. The author, however, opposes this theory, because if the position of the marking screw is correct, it means that the plugs are still there.

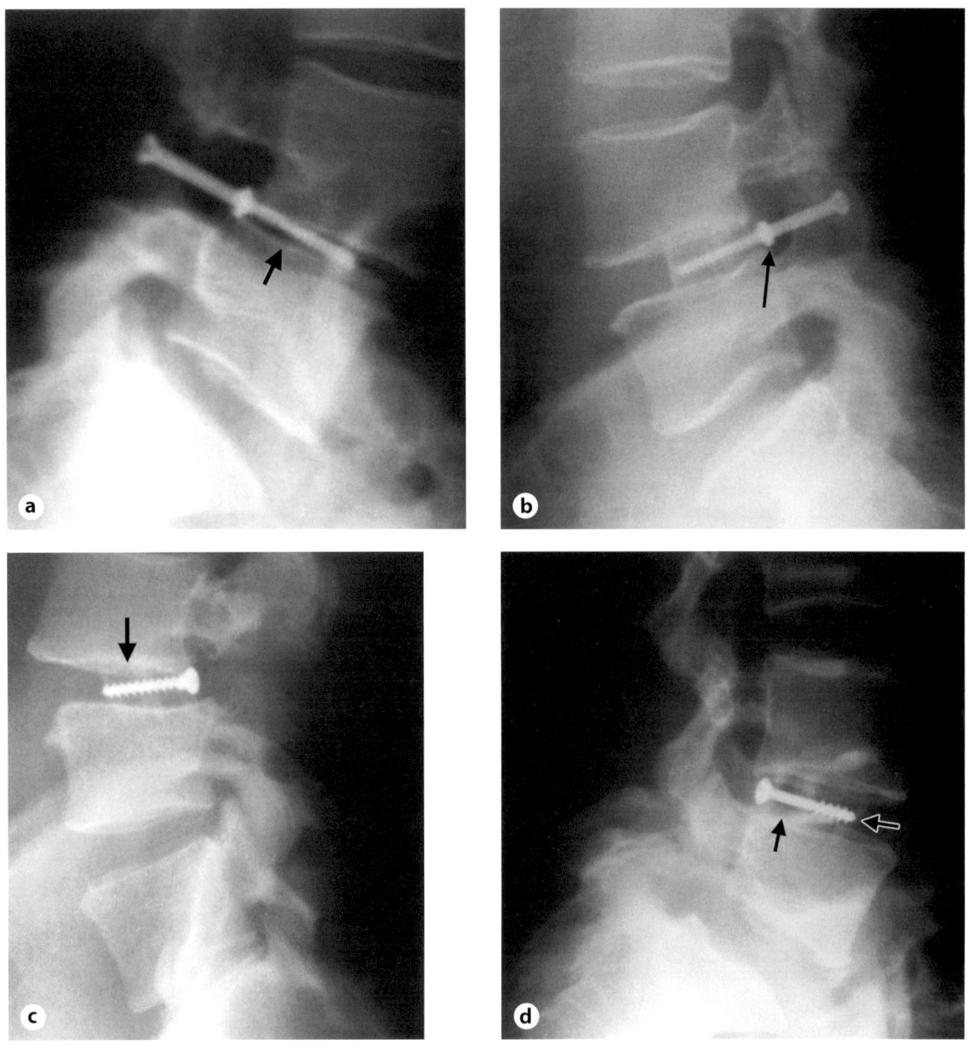

Fig. 89. a Both plugs are not visible. **b** Plugs are visible. **c** Only ventral plug is visible. **d** Dorsal plug is visible.

Unexpected Effects

- Dislocation of the plugs
- Wrong direction of the plugs
- No compact fusion
- Technical interference
- Mal- or non-union

Slippage of the dorsal plug! It occurs under unstable technical condition (the plug is not optimally located in a compact fashion) only the dorsal plug can slip into the spinal canal in the dorsal direction.

Plug Dislocation

There are two kinds of plugs slippage:

(a) Dorsal slippage type (fig. 90)

(b) Fixed plugs – dorsolateral slippage (fig. 91)

Cases

Last check shows that the dorsal plug slipped to dorsal area. Patient did not complain about pain.

Four weeks postoperatively, X-ray shows that the ventral and dorsal plugs slipped together into the spinal canal, even though the patient felt no pain because the plug is lying free between the upper and lower nerve roots (fig. 91a, b).

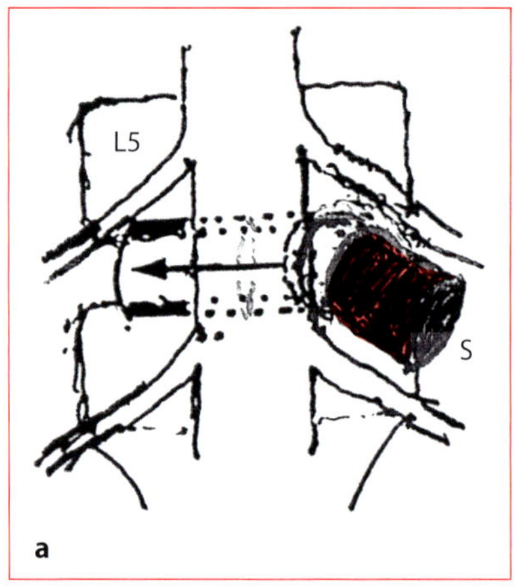

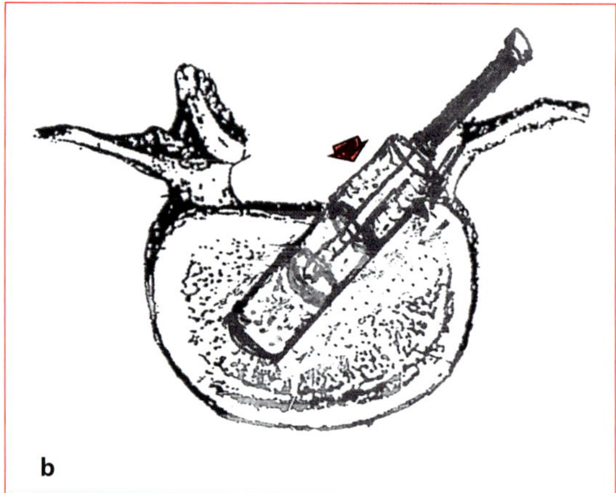

Fig. 90. a, b Dorsal plug is slipping (S) into the spinal canal.

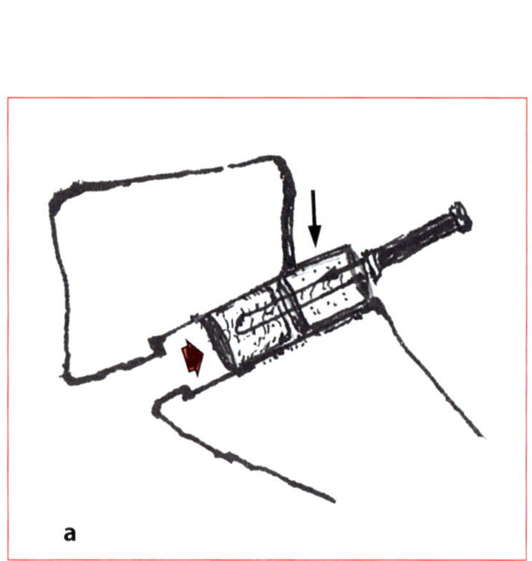

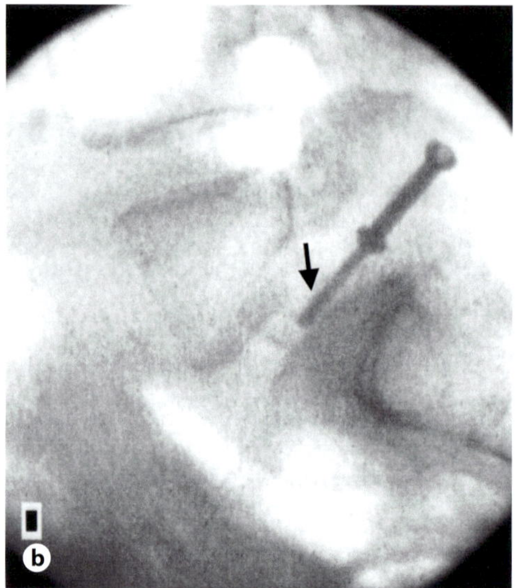

Fig. 91. a, b Fixed bone plugs slipping together.

Wrong Direction

One case shows a screw which goes in the wrong direction. Identified postoperatively during routine check (fig. 92). The reason may be that the patient has a strong lumbar sacral kyphosis.

Postoperative routine check shows optimal fit of the posterior plug in the intervertebral space (fig. 92).

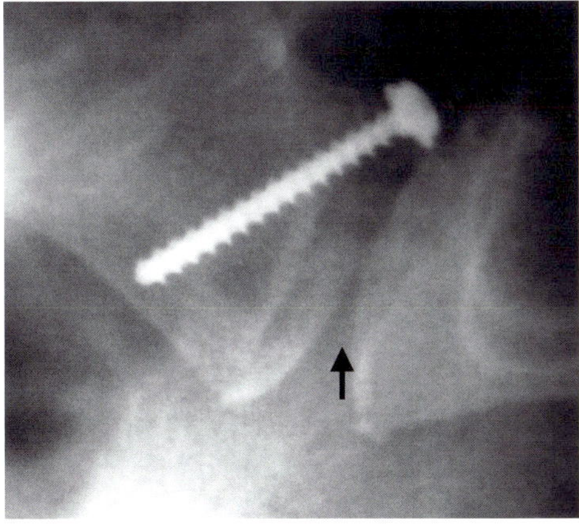

Fig. 92. Wrong direction. Screw is located well for the dorsal plug.

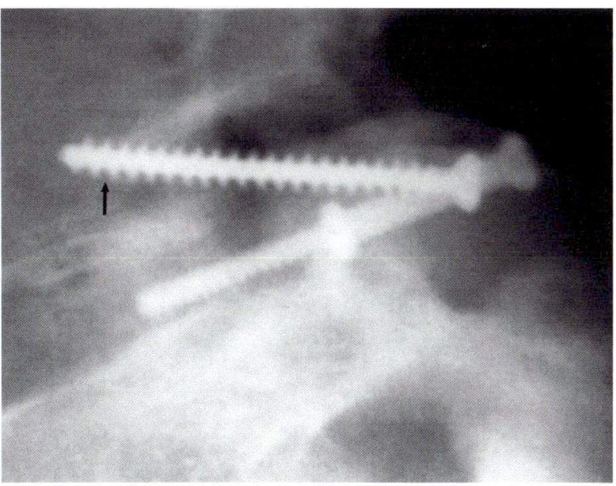

Fig. 93. Additional protection for plugs fixed with a normal screw in the vertebral column.

Technical Interferences

One other case shows the fixed screw is not placed in the centre and lies in an upper position in the plugs (fig. 94a, b). The dorsal plug is ideally located and it produces no side effects, resulting in a satisfactory outcome.

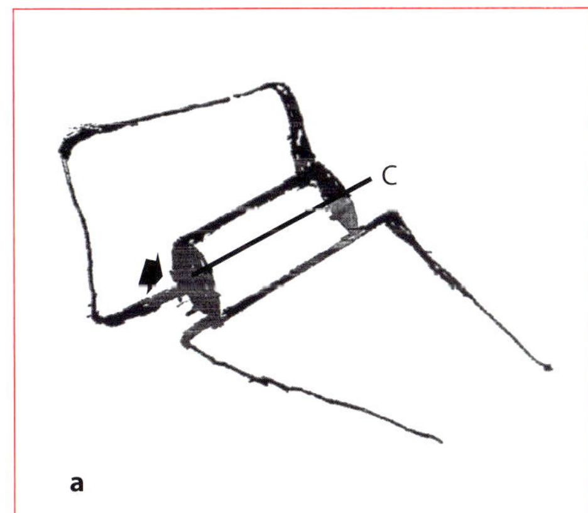

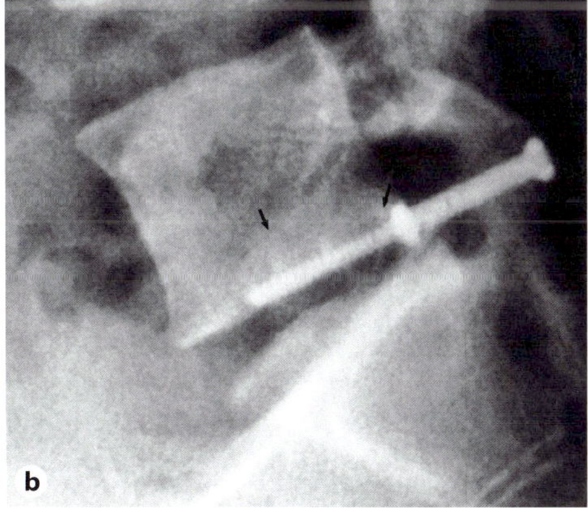

Fig. 94. a, b Drilled uppermost part of the intervertebral space. C = Center of plugs.

Comment

Preoperative lumbar mobility shows that the patient has an extreme hypermobility (as in acrobats).

Intraoperative check confirmed that no compact fitting of the plugs by fusion had taken place. Radiological check shows that the plugs were dislocated. An additional screw was fixated for stabilization (fig. 93).

Mal- or Non-Union

CT lumbar shows partially nonfused plugs, especially caudal part of plugs (fig. 95). The author has had no experience of mal- or non-union.

Case

In this case, the author suspected a mal-union of the caudal part, for which reason the patient was off work for 6 months. During the same time the treatment was the wearing of a lumbar corset. The patient is now very happy, free of pain, and enjoys sports like skiing, mountain biking, snowboarding, etc.

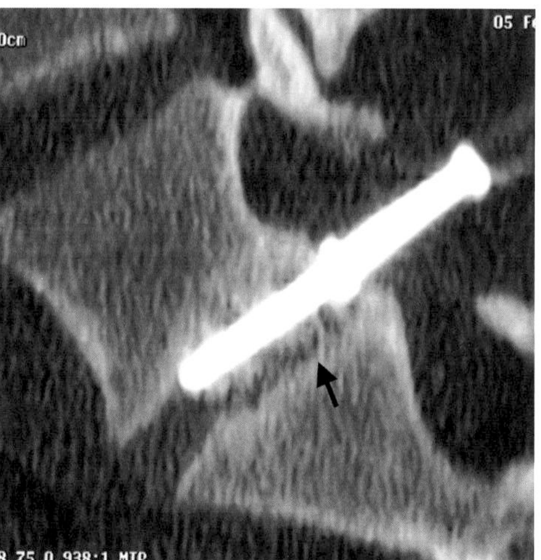

Fig. 95. Upperside shows compact ossifying of plug and vertebra body, and lower side shows incomplete fusion.

Discussion

A wide variety of methods has been used in the past few decades for surgical treatment with foreign bodies' fixation for lumbar instability such as: posterior-ventral screw fixation, plate/screw fixation, exclusively ventral approaches and combined ventral and dorsal approaches. In recent years, cages made of titanium, carbon composite, or PEEK, with or without a hydroxyapatite coating and with or without autologous spongiosa filling, have been increasingly used for interbody support. In all these techniques, regardless of whether support is achieved by the cage alone or with use of additional instrumentation, foreign substances are employed (fig. 96a).

Since there were no reliably safe operations available for fusion for lumbar instability without the use of foreign substances, the author began his own bone fusion technique in 1990, a technique which guarantees good stability without use of a foreign substance.

The surgical transplantation-fusion technique involving the UOPIF procedure leads in most cases to good stabilization and allows immediate mobilization. However, the screw and plate implantation fixation systems employed as well as the cages themselves constitute foreign substances. Chronic foreign body reactions are possible when foreign substances are used, even if such reactions are generally denied at present. In addition, the costs of the implants are considerable.

All things considered, the present technique utilizing autologous bone plugs represents one of the most simple, compact, safe and cost-effective fusion procedures for stabilization of the lumbar spine (fig. 96b).

A great advantage of this approach is the use of a living plug of material taken from the patient's own body small in scale and yet very effective. Furthermore, it has an important function in the body center.

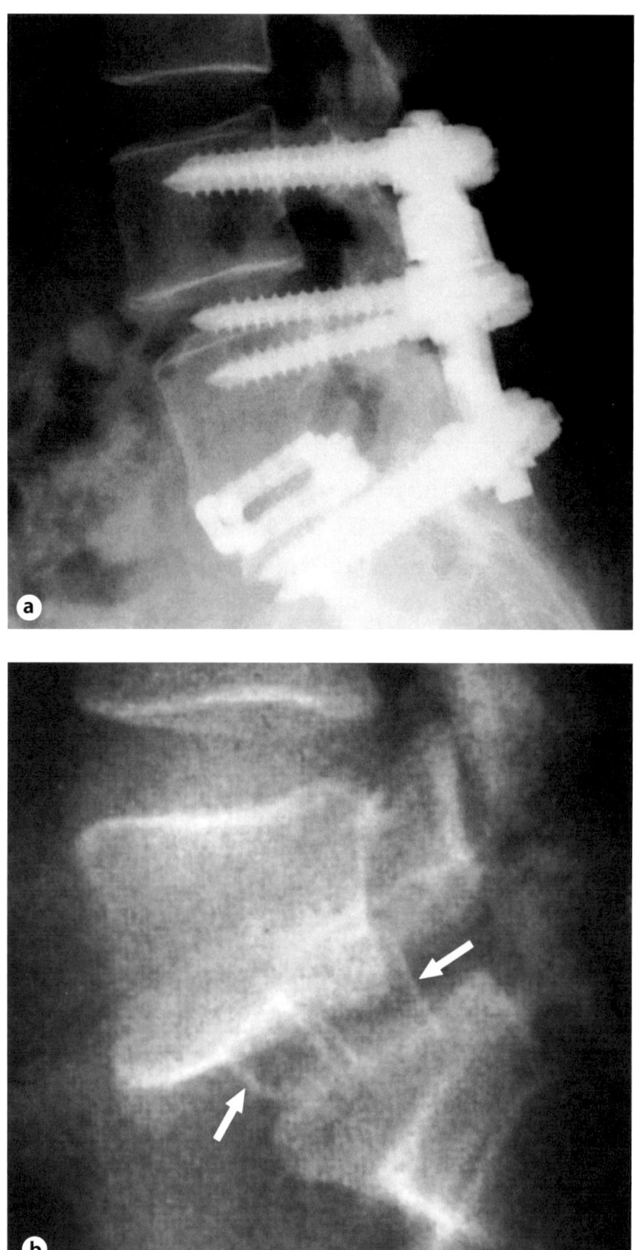

Fig. 96. a Implant fixation. **b** Transplant fusion.

History of Transplantation Surgery

Transplantation procedures have been reported from the 9th century BC, according to the literature, being performed as an experimental procedure on animals.

1878, human-to-human transplantation, but not with autologous material.

1881, skin graft.

Throughout history, people have always been intrigued by the possibilities of transplantation of organs and tissues from one body to another. During the 15th century, we can find references in the historical medical literature of attempted blood transfusions as well as the transplantation of teeth (presumably from cadavers). A skin transplant and a corneal transplant were reported in medical journals dating as far back as 1880. Of course, these early attempts at transplantation were usually unsuccessful. It was not until early in the 20th century that transplantation offered the promise of renewed health and life envisioned by our ancestors.

1906, first corneal transplant by Austrian ophthalmologist Dr. Edward Zinn.

1908, first skin allograft by Swiss Surgeon Jacques Louis Reverdin.

1911, initial use of homologous vein tissue in arterial reconstruction.

1949, establishment of US Navy Tissue Bank.

1954, first successful live kidney transplantation from identical twins performed by Dr. Joseph Murray and Dr. David Hume in Boston, Mass., USA. The recipient had normal kidney function for 8 years.

1963, first liver transplant performed by Dr. Thomas Starzl.

1963, first lung transplant performed by Dr. James Hardy at the University of Mississippi Medical Center, Jackson, Miss., USA.

1967, first heart transplant performed by Dr. Christian Barnard at Grote Shure Hospital, South Africa. The recipient had normal heart function for 19 months.

1971, introduction of cryopreserved human skin allografts.

1972, The Uniform Anatomical Gift Act establishes the Uniform Organ Donor Card as a legal document in all 50 states making it possible for anyone 18 years or older to legally donate his or her organs upon death.

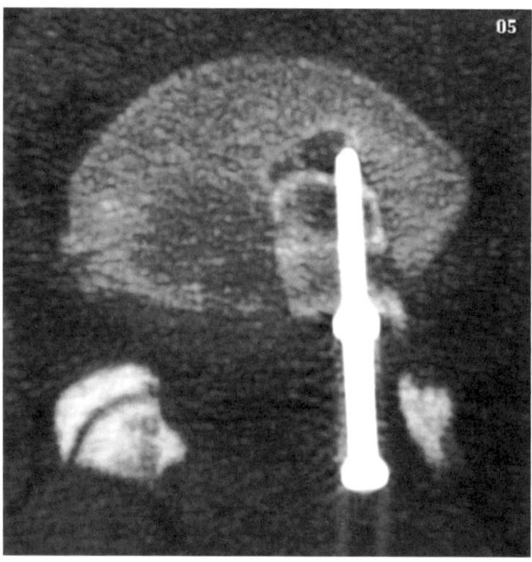

Fig. 97. 1990, first lumbar autologous bone plug fusion.

1984, National Organ Transplant Act (NOTA) establishes a nationwide computer registry operated by the United Network for Organ Sharing (UNOS); authorizes financial support for Organ Procurement Organizations (OPOs); prohibits buying and selling of organs in the US.

1986, required request laws stipulate that hospitals develop policies to identify patients as potential donors and approach families about organ donation.

1988, FDA approves Viaspan which greatly extends the preservation of donated livers.

1989, first successful live liver transplantation.

1990, autologous lumbar bone plugs fusion (unilateral oblique posterior interbody fusion (UOPIF) by the author: S. Oh) performed, Switzerland. CT pictures after fusion show living plugs (fig. 97).

The history of transplantation is one of an epic journey describing the medical community's quest to understand how the human body works and its most daring efforts to defy illness and death. Between the lines, too powerful to capture in words, are its most important components – the generosity of organ and tissue donors, and the courage of transplant recipients.

The extraordinary human and medical progress depicted here, accelerating in recent decades, is taking us forward to a world in which we can help each other in ways that previous generations could never imagine.

Presentations and Publications

Presentations

The first fusion operation was performed in November 1990. Four years later in 1994, the author presented the bone plugs fusion procedure at the Swiss Surgical Congress at Lucerne (Switzerland). Since then the operation has been presented at several international congresses and universities (table 4).

There were also four presentations at several universities in Seoul and Pusan/South Korea in May 2004.

Publications

See table 4.

Comment

The frontispiece of the Journal of Korean Neurosurgical Society 2003, the volume of which demonstrates the operative technical note for plugs fusion operation, is shown in figure 98. Figures 99–103 are certificates presented to Prof. Dr. Oh in appreciation of his work.

Table 4. Summary of presentations and publications

a The new operation technique presentations:

- Lucerne 'Swiss Surgical Union-Congress', 1994
- Berlin '10th European Congress of Neurosurgery', 1995
- Seoul/Korea 'Congress of Neurosurgery', 1995
- Saragoza/Spain 'European Spinal Congress', 1997
- Amsterdam '11th International Congress of Neurosurgery', 1997
- Lausanne 'Swiss Surgical Union Congress', 1998
- Berlin '1st World Spine Congress', 2000
- Seoul/Korea 'Congress of Neurosurgery', 2000
- Seoul/Korea 'Presentation Korea University' 2000 (fig. 103)
- Pusan/Korea, 'Presentation at In-Jae University', 2004 (fig. 102)
- Seoul/Korea, 'Presentation Korea University', 2004 (fig. 100)
- Seoul/Korea 'Presentation at Chung-An University', 2004 (fig. 101)

b Publications of the new operation technique

- Knochenzapfen Spondylodese bei lumbarem Wirbelgleiten. Informierte Arzt, 1999;20:409–414.
- Spondylodese mittels Knochenzapfen. Medical Tribune 1999, No. 39.
- Bone plugs fusion for treatment for lumbar spondylolisthesis. Berlin, World Spine, 2000, pp 753–760.
- Oblique posterior interbody fusion with bone plugs by unilateral approach for treatment of lumbar instability – Technical note. J Korean Neurosurg Soc, 2003:33 (fig. 99).

Print ISSN 1225-8245
On-line ISSN 1598-7876
On-line. www.neurosurgery.or.kr

JOURNAL OF
KOREAN NEUROSURGICAL
SOCIETY

대한신경외과학회지

May 2003
Vol 33 No 5

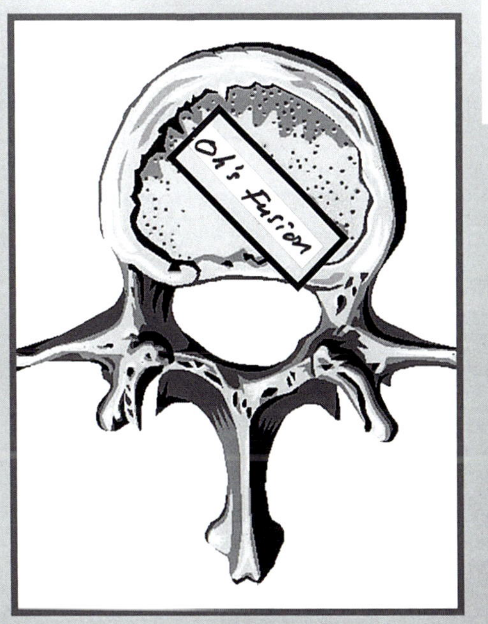

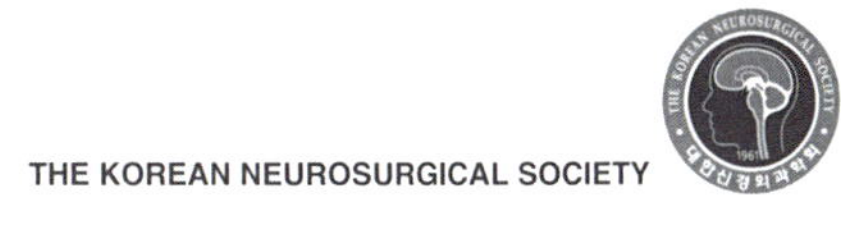

Fig. 98. Frontispiece of the *Journal of Korean Neurosurgical Society* 2003.

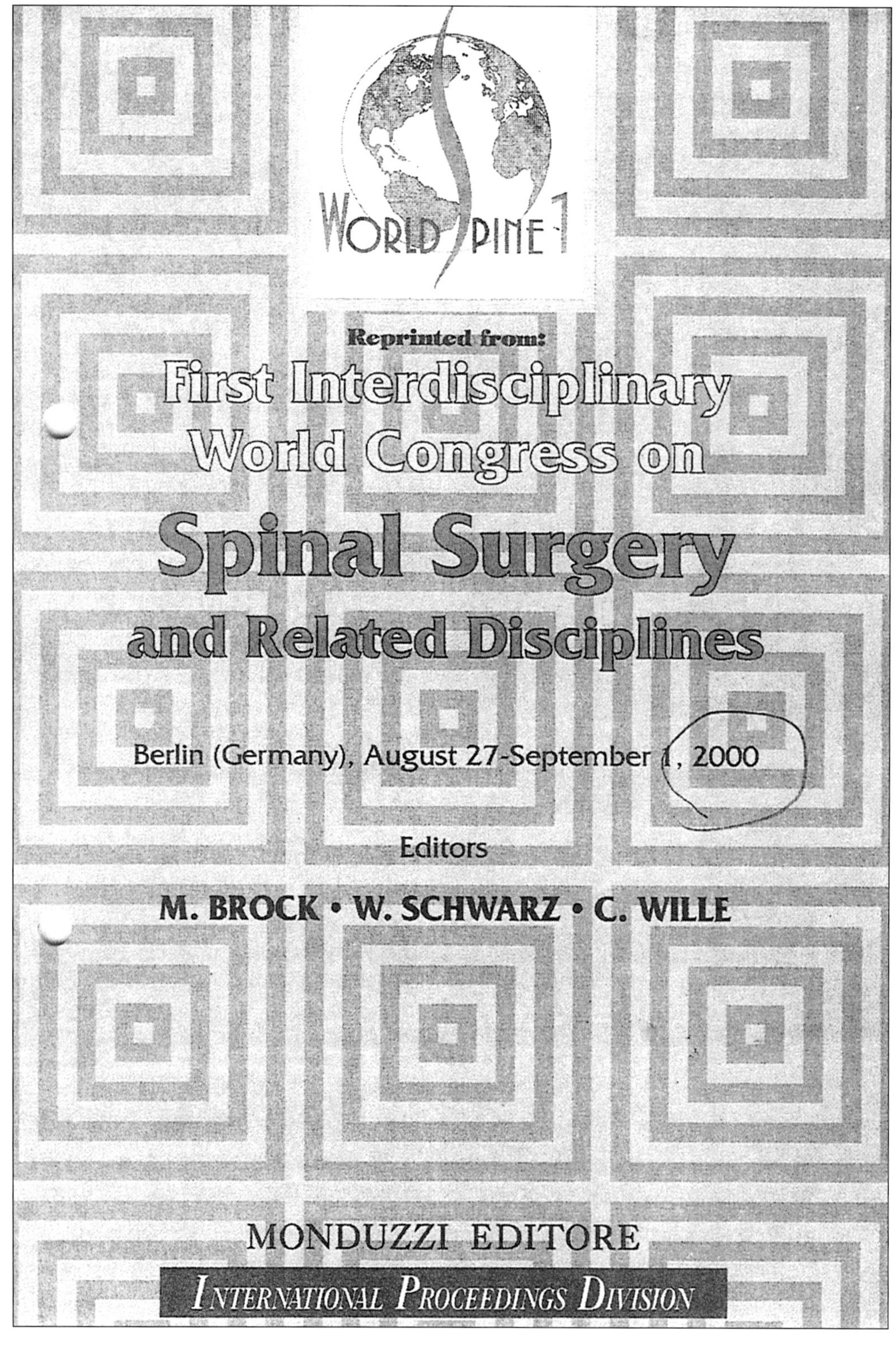

Fig. 99. Cover of the proceedings program.

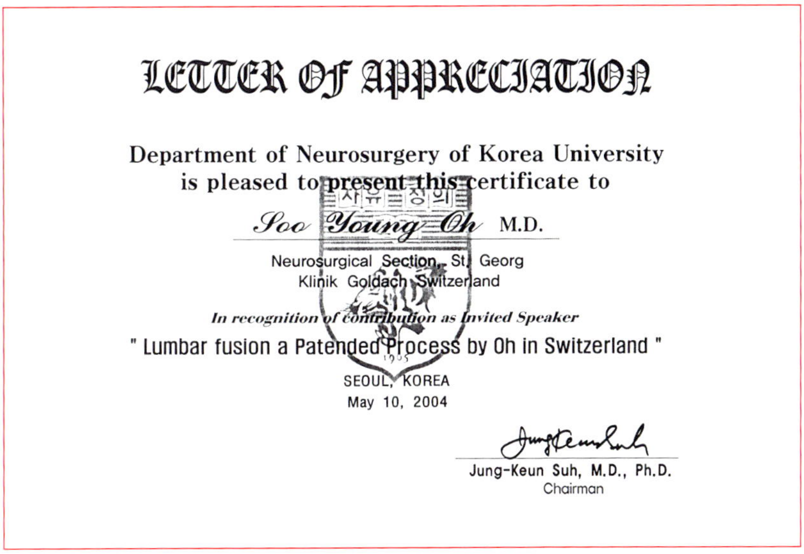

LETTER OF APPRECIATION

Department of Neurosurgery of Korea University
is pleased to present this certificate to

Soo Young Oh M.D.

Neurosurgical Section, St. Georg
Klinik Goldach Switzerland

In recognition of contribution as Invited Speaker

" Lumbar fusion a Patended Process by Oh in Switzerland "

SEOUL, KOREA
May 10, 2004

Jung-Keun Suh, M.D., Ph.D.
Chairman

Fig. 100. Presentation Korea University, Seoul/Korea.

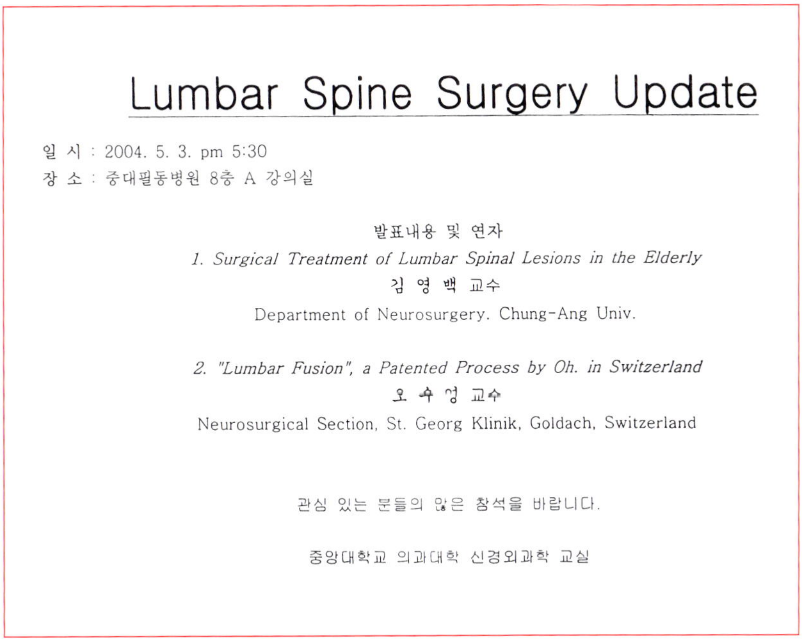

Lumbar Spine Surgery Update

일 시 : 2004. 5. 3. pm 5:30
장 소 : 중대필동병원 8층 A 강의실

발표내용 및 연자

1. Surgical Treatment of Lumbar Spinal Lesions in the Elderly
김 영 백 교수
Department of Neurosurgery. Chung-Ang Univ.

2. "Lumbar Fusion", a Patented Process by Oh. in Switzerland
오 수 영 교수
Neurosurgical Section, St. Georg Klinik, Goldach, Switzerland

관심 있는 분들의 많은 참석을 바랍니다.

중앙대학교 의과대학 신경외과학 교실

Fig. 101. Presentation Chung-Ang University, Seoul/Korea.

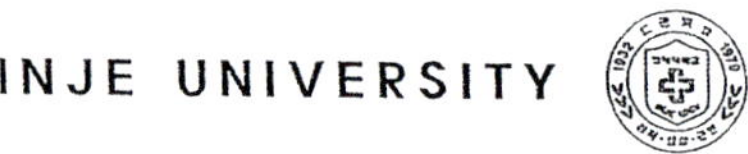

INJE UNIVERSITY

May 19, 2004

Letter of Certificate

This is to certify that

Dr. med. Soo-Young Oh
Spezialarzt FMH fur Neurochirurgie
Grabenstrasse 47
7000 Chur, Switzerland

has given a lecture to graduate students, faculty and regional specialisst of spine surgery with title of

「Posterior Interbody Fusion with Bone Plugs for Treatment of Lumber Instability」

on May 11, 2004 at lecture hall 1.

Prof. Key-Yong KIM, M.D., Ph.D
Dean, College of Medicine
Inje University
633 Kaegum-dong, busanjin-ku,
Busan, Korea

Fig. 102. Presentation Inje University, Busan/Korea.

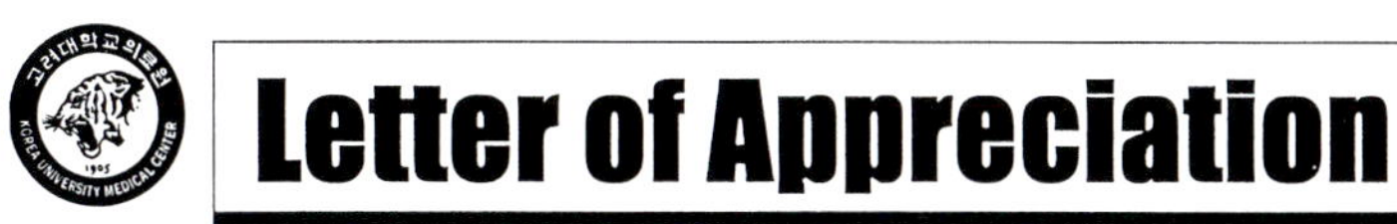

Oh, Soo Young, M.D.
Clinical Professor

On behalf of staff members & alumni of Department of Neurosurgery, Korea University, Medical College we would like to express our sincere thanks hereby for giving us lecture entitled;

"Bone plugs fusion for treatment of lumbar spondylolisthesis".

As in the past, it is always honor to have you as our clinical professor and we thank you for your tremendous contribution to our department. In witness whereof, this letter of appreciation will be awarded to you.

September 29, 2000

Department of Neurosurgery, Medical College, Korea University

Jung Keun Suh, M.D., Ph.D.
Professor and Chairman

Fig. 103. Presentation Korea University, Seoul/Korea.

Individual Remarks

The author had an idea in his mind which was realized with the development of the lumbar fusion operation with pelvis bone transplants to the instable lumbar column. He had had experience with cervical fusion with bone plugs for many years with good results.

The realization of this medical project was all brought about by his own efforts. The beginning was difficult, also in the necessity to keep faith with colleagues and insurance bodies, always to explain his methods and actions and the reasons for them, and which advantages the operation has in comparison to others.

On the other hand, it was the huge success of this operation and the satisfaction from the patients' side which gave him the strength and encouragement to go forward.

A decisive step was the acknowledgement from the Swiss Government; Oh's operation was taken up in the list for health care.

Patient Activity

Over 60 former patients have established a group called 'Aktionskomitee'. They support the author's living plug procedure (translation):

Action Committee
Bone Plug Transplant-Fusion Operation
Markus Derrer
Casa Scardanal
CH–7016 Trin Mulin (Switzerland)
Tel. 081 635 18 08, Fax 079 610 64 22

BSV
Federal Board of Social Insurance
Application for ELK
c/o Dr. med. Felix Gurtner
Effingerstrasse 20
CH–3003 Bern (Switzerland)

Chur, June 16, 2003

Dear Dr. Gurtner,

As members of the board of the committee 'Pro Fusion without Metal', and as patients previously operated on by Prof. Dr. med. S. Oh, we would like to elucidate the situation from our point of view.

Markus Derrer, Trin Mulin: Most of us were operated on by other surgeons/ orthopedists on one or several occasions before we were treated by Prof. Dr. Oh. In most of the cases, however, these previous treatments did not have the intended long-term success.

As a private patient, I was operated on for two herniated discs in 1989 and 1990 by 'very reputable' surgeons without success. Thus, I not only had to give up my career as a military and civil pilot, but would also still be living more or less as a fully disabled person to this day. Through a lucky coincidence, during my time of complete helplessness (after the two operations), Prof. Oh and his fusion method was recommended to me through one of his former patients, and, because of this, I now enjoy a high quality of life.

And it does not end there. The costs of health insurance and disabled allowance would by now have amounted to approximately CHF 1.5 million. An alternative might have been a major orthopedic surgical intervention including the fitting of metal rods for stabilization of the spine. In their complete helplessness, the consultants recommended this to me as being the only way. Thank God I did not consent to these suggestions, as with that method, I would still be suffering today, as I know from many cases.

Ueli Möller, Chur: After suffering for a long time, our son Ueli (born Feb. 24, 1987) had his spine operated on by Prof. Dr. S. Oh in November 2002. The method used by Prof. Oh proved, in comparison to other more established methods, to be most efficient.

Through the use of bone material from his own body, a well-developed technique, and excellent care, Ueli was able to leave hospital after a very short time.

Today, Ueli is in perfect health. He lives completely free of pain and has fully recovered his original mobility.

Thanks to the method used by Prof. Oh, on July 28, 2003 Ueli will be able to begin his long planned apprenticeship as joiner without any noteworthy constraints. Thanks to Prof. Oh's method, the in part very discouraging prognoses of other doctors did not come true.

For our son, this method of operation has opened up a completely new perspective for his future.

From our point of view as tax payers, premium payers (SWICA health insurance) and as closely involved people (parents), we are convinced that the method used by Prof. S. Oh is an ingenious idea that offers many tangible advantages:

(1) Through the use of bone material obtained from the patient themselves there are *no additional costs* for expensive implants.

(2) Shorter lengths of treatment and convalescence result in *much reduced costs*.

(3) A much more *'humane'* treatment, as the patient is spared the known side effects caused by foreign bodies (titanium implants) and unnecessary long surgical interventions.

It would, therefore, be a true advance for us all if, thanks to an early recognition of this method of treatment, many future patients were given the possibility to live a pain- and worry-free future through the Oh operation technique. We are happy to provide you with further detailed information from the viewpoint of the patients.

Yours sincerely
Board of Action Committee

Markus Derrer, Trin Mulin

Luzius Parpan, Chur

Rolf + Marianne Möller, Chur
Parents

Ueli Möller
Patient

cc. Prof. Dr. S. Oh, Chur

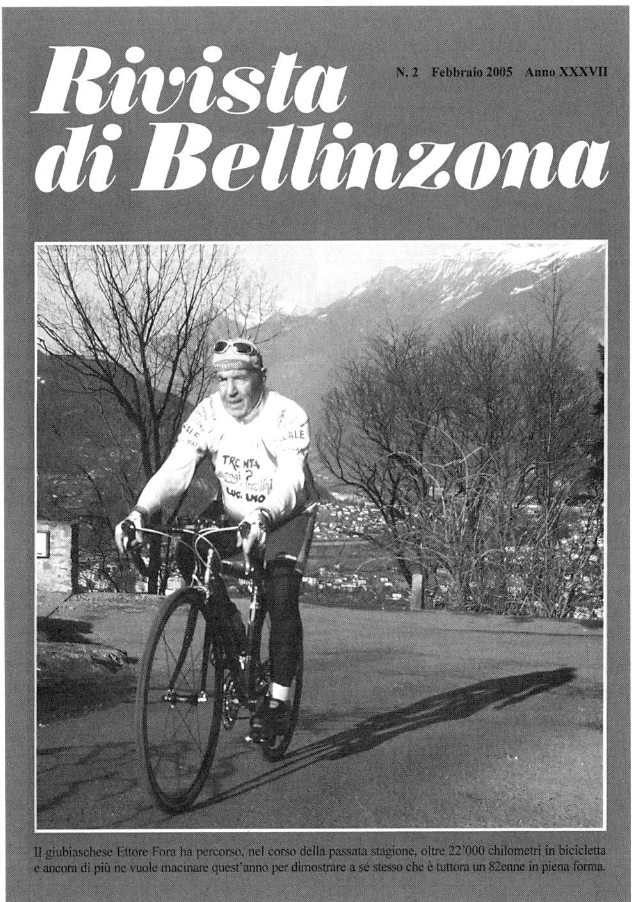

Rivista di Bellinzona

N. 2 Febbraio 2005 Anno XXXVII

Il giubiaschese Ettore Fora ha percorso, nel corso della passata stagione, oltre 22'000 chilometri in bicicletta e ancora di più ne vuole macinare quest'anno per dimostrare a sé stesso che è tuttora un 82enne in piena forma.

Fig. 104–107. Pictures from patients showing how they can enjoy sports like skiing, mountain-biking and hunting again thanks to Oh's fusion procedure.

Thankful patients have sent Prof. Oh pictures to show him how they can enjoy sports like skiing, mountain-biking and hunting.

- An 84-year-old patient wrote him postcards to let him know that he biked 80,000 km after the operation (the operation was performed when he was 76 years old) (fig. 104).
- The youngest patient came when he was 15 years old (he wrote his account of his experiences himself which is here enclosed). He now enjoys skiing and hunting (fig. 105a, b).
- Another young patient now pursues extreme mountain biking (fig. 106).
- One patient was an airline pilot prior to his illness. After his 2nd lumbar operation he was no longer able to work and was in receipt of payment from a disabled persons pension. following appointments with the author and treatment with Oh's fusion procedure, he feels healthy and is very satisfied at being 100% fit for work again. He is now president of the 'Aktionskomitee' for Oh's fusion operation (fig. 107).

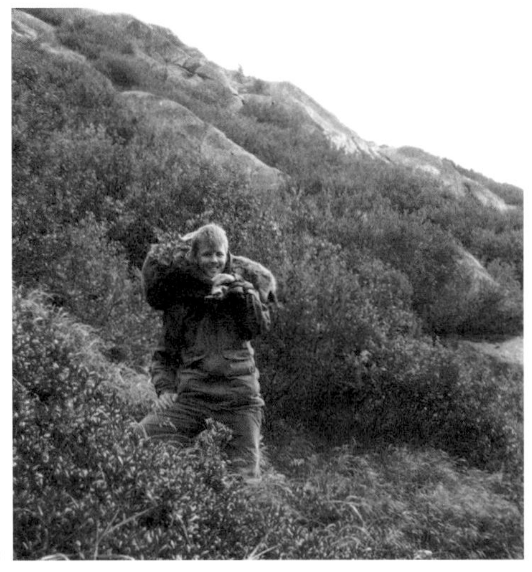
105a

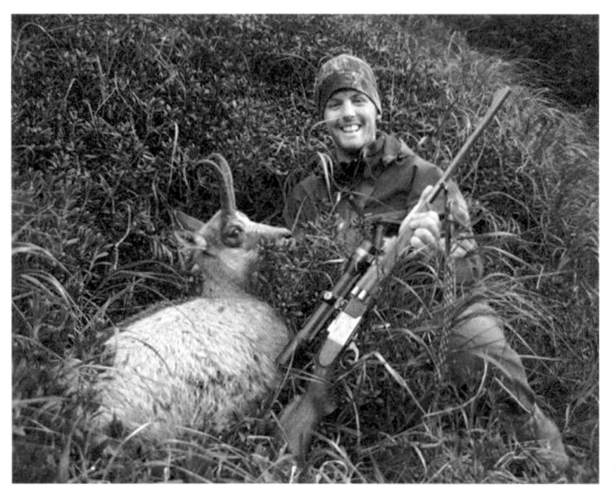
105b

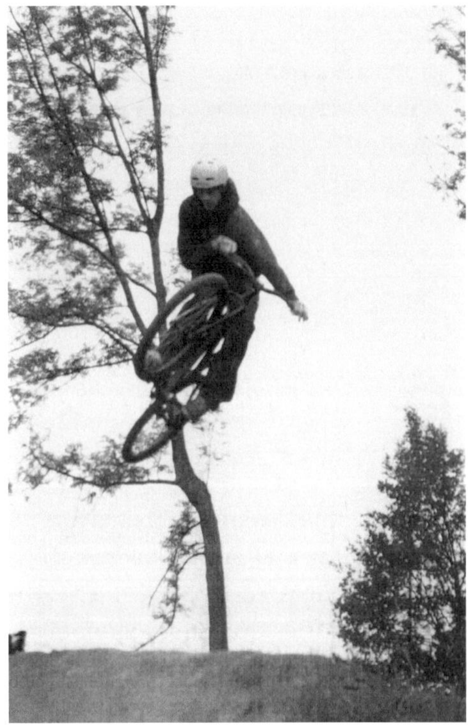
106

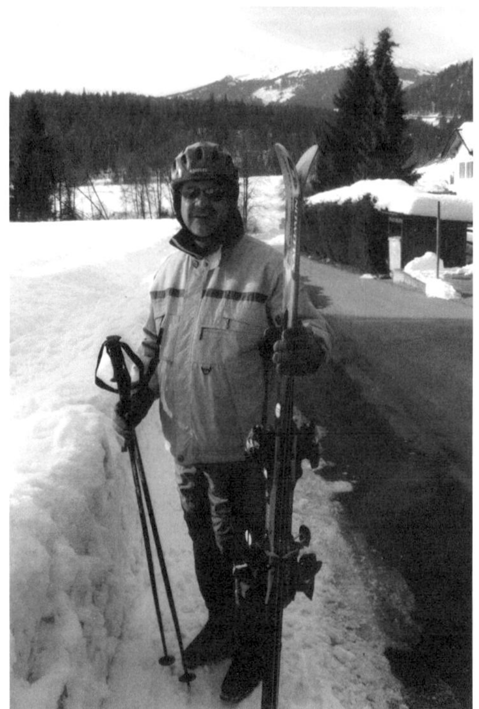
107

Report and Memories of My Back Pains by Ueli Möller

On Monday morning after a mountain hike in September of 2002, I suddenly felt strong pains in the lower half of my back. I did not think much of it, as I had already experienced pain sometimes after cycling; these pains, however, normally disappeared after 2 days at most if I watched my movements and rested a bit. So I continued to go to school for this and the following week. The pain, however, did not subside, indeed it grew stronger. On Monday morning, 2 weeks after I had felt the pain for the first time, I was hardly able to get up anymore. I had such shooting pains in the lower part of my back that I could only walk bent over and I felt the need to lie down as much as possible. Now, I also started to ask myself what that thing was, which was jutting out down on my back. I contacted the Swica Health Center and was able to go to the doctor on Tuesday morning. He examined the area and took me straight to get my back X-rayed from the front and the side and asked me to wait for the results of the images. Doctor Beer, the physician, stood there with a ruler and measured the distance of the displacement. It was 8 mm. We then returned to his office and he asked me some questions. He sent me home with pain killers and medicines for relaxation of the muscles.

Over the following weeks, I had to return about three times a week to the Swica health center for physiotherapy sessions with Andreiko Knappe. It did not help much. Whatever we achieved during the therapy sessions was undone through the long periods of sitting or standing at school. Even the therapist was of the opinion that this approach did not make any sense. However, the therapist and the doctors kept talking all the time about building up muscles and strengthening the back, so that I could live with a displaced vertebra. They said that an operation would only be needed in an extreme case. Nobody mentioned that I had a very unstable spine and that further displacements could occur. For me the situation seemed hopeless. Everything that I had looked forward to over the next years was destroyed. I simply let life go by and became more and more withdrawn and pensive.

In the end, the doctor did send me for one more examination with Dr. M. at the Cantonal Hospital. It became clear that it was necessary to operate, as it would never be right otherwise. He explained to me that I would receive two rods, six screws and three cages into and around my spine. I was told that there would be no alternative or other possibility for me. We again returned to his office and he asked me some questions. Among other things he asked me what I, as a person just about to go into professional education, was planning to do in 2003. I told him that I wanted to become a carpenter and that I had already found a place for my apprenticeship. He merely answered: 'You can forget about it. You will never be able to do such an apprenticeship with this kind of displacement. Sport and any excessive strain of your back are also forbidden to you!' My whole world was turned upside down, I almost collapsed. The last thing I wanted to become was a person with such an amount of metal in his back that he is attracted by magnets. This is how I imagined myself in those first moments.

We were asked by Dr. M. to book for a further appraisal of my back at the Schulthess Clinic in Zurich. Although we did this immediately on 11/11/2002, it took the Schulthess Clinic 9 days – in this very sensitive time for me – to inform me that I had an appointment with Prof. G. for an examination on 22/01/2003. We were told to register with the IV (social payments for the disabled) Branch, Chur, for a disabled allowance.

However, for a more exact diagnosis, to see how much the discs had been damaged and what exactly would happen, I had to go to the Cantonal Hospital of Chur on a Wednesday morning at 6 o'clock for a computer tomography. I had to lay in a tube for about 20 min and was played some music.

During these weeks my parents and I sought a second opinion from Dr. Martin Stetter, who we know very well privately, and he confirmed everything.

During this time my father said that Silvia Derrer from Trin Mulin near Flims had told him that her father had had similar problems, but that he had been operated on by a Prof. Oh. She urged my father not to do anything and told her father about it. He invited us for dinner that same evening and told us his long tale of woe and his eventual healing through an operation by Prof. Oh. Following that evening we contacted Prof. Oh and obtained an appointment. My father obtained the X-ray and computer tomography images and brought them to him. The first time I came to his surgery, I was surprised to see such a small man and was somewhat concerned. However, when he started to talk to me and examined me, I realized that this man knew what he was doing and only wanted what was best for me. I also preferred his way of operating to the options with the screws. He told me that I was his youngest patient but that it was necessary to operate nonetheless. However, I would recover very quickly, as I was so young. I had about three sessions with him. After that we established the date for the operation. This was for the second week of November in the Marienfried Clinic in Niederuzwil. I decided to take the operate as quickly as I did as this was the only way I would have been healthy enough to start my apprenticeship. I did this in spite of advice to the contrary from the Swica, the Cantonal Hospital and Dr. S.

I tried to prepare myself for the operation. There was no problem from my school, they simply sent me my homework.

The operation took place on a Tuesday. When I woke up, my parents were sitting at my bedside. I could only lift my thumb and ask them: 'Is everything ok with me and you?' Then I fell asleep again. I did not feel any pain at this point. That only came at night. I needed many painkiller injections. It was an ordeal and I had to suffer a lot. But I came through it. At the beginning I was not even able to turn in bed and had to call the nurses for help. I found that very embarrassing and also the fact that I had to learn again how to get up and how to walk properly. On the third day after the operation, the professor called me and told me that I was allowed to go home. I was very surprised. I had expected 3 weeks and now this! He explained to me that this was possible because he had his surgery in Chur and so it would be easy for me to come for examinations.

So, I traveled home in the VW bus of my parents. The car was well padded and I was able to lie on my back, however, this caused me a lot of pain and I was happy when we finally reached home. I appreciated being allowed to recover in my own home. All my friends came to visit me and were very supportive. I was also grateful to my parents who kept forcing me to do my exercises. I had to learn everything from scratch. Walking, standing properly, but most of the time I lay in bed. It was hard to wait to be able to sit again. I was only allowed to lie or to stand. In the end I got used to everything.

The whole operation went smoothly and I am really grateful for that.

In April came the second operation in which the screw that was marking the planted screw was removed. It only took 1 day and was nothing in comparison to what I had had to endure up to then.

I thank everyone who supported me during this time. It is important to me to fight for this method to be recognized all over the world, as I and indeed many other patients were allowed to experience its effectiveness on their own body!

The most important part of all this is that on August 4th, 2003, I was able to begin my apprenticeship as a joiner – an occupation that is known for the fact that one has to lift a lot. I can even do all the sports that I was doing before the start of my back problems. These are for example: cycling, hiking, skating, snowboarding, skiing, etc…! And the best part of it – it is all pain-free!

Bonaduz, November 30, 2003

Ueli Möller

Conclusion

Over the last 18 years, the author has individually treated about 200 patients with lumbar instability.

- All patients were observed individually.
- Postoperative clinical checks were done for a duration of about a few months and some patients had long-term observation.
- The plugs with compact vertebral column osseous consolidation look as strong as normal segmental columns.
- Autologous plugs ossified the 'block' lumbar spine column.
- No foreign materials are used.
- No reactions due to foreign body or complications.
- 3E criteria of good fusion method. Acknowledgement by the Swiss Government.
- Living plugs function without any change to their biological nature. Effectiveness.
- The alternative to transplantation with bone from the patient's own body is a treatment with spine fusion.
- First book published internationally on this method.

Acknowledgement

The author is indebted to the Governments of the Canton of Graubünden and the capital of Graubünden, Chur, Switzerland, for sponsoring this book.

Thanks to Further Sponsors:

- Clinic Marienfried, Schams Hossein, MD, Niederuzwil, Switzerland
- Clinic St. Georg, Hutter Beda, Goldach, Switzerland
- Embassy of the Republic of Korea, Berne, Switzerland
- Federation of Korean Association, Switzerland
- Graf Hans Rudolf, Küssnacht, Switzerland
- Habeil-Oh Helena, Muri, BE, Switzerland
- Kim Yong-Kie, Neurosurgeon, Vista, Calif., USA
- Korean Senior Club, Switzerland
- Korean Artists Association in Switzerland
- Kunz Bruno, MD, Medical Advisor, St. Gallen, Switzerland
- Oh-Graf Christine, Chur, Switzerland
- Oh Eduard, Thalwil, Switzerland
- Oh Jacqueline, Chur, Switzerland
- Woo Young-In, Gümligen, Switzerland
- Wyss Ursula, Sargans, Switzerland

Thanks for assistance (recommendation) for the acknowledgments of this operation technique to:

- Augustin Vincent, Dr. iur., lawyer, santésuisse Graubünden, Chur, Switzerland
- de Haller Jacques, MD, President FMH, Swiss Medical Association, Bern, Switzerland
- Derrrer Markus, President Aktionskomitee, Trin/GR, Switzerland
- Evangelista Mario, eidg. dipl. Krankenversicherungs-Experte, Chur, Switzerland
- Hablützel Martin, Schoolmaster, St. Gallen, Switzerland
- Indra Peter, MD, Medical Manager, (Ex-)Helsana Insurance, Zürich Switzerland
- Janom-Steiner Barbara, Regierungsrätin of Canton Graubünden, Chur, Switzerland
- Jung Keun Suh, Dept. Neurosurgery, Korea University, Seoul/Korea
- Kim Ki-Young, MD Prof., Dean, In-Jae medical College, Pusan, Korea
- Kim Young-Baeg MD Prof., Dept. Neurosurgery, College of Medicine, Chung-An Univ. Seoul/Korea
- Kunz Rudolf, Dr. iur, HSG, Lawyer LL.M., Chur, Switzerland
- Möller Rolf, Member Aktionskomitee, Bonaduz/GR, Switzerland
- Portmann Théo, Dr. iur., lawyer, Chur, Switzerland
- Portner Carlo, Dr. iur., lawyer, CEO Aerzteverein GR, Chur, Switzerland
- Seiler Rolf, MD Prof. Neurosurgeon, Ex-Director Dept. Neurosurgery school of medicine, Univ. Berne, Switzerland
- Sgier Alfred, MD, Neurosurgeon, Hirslanden Clinic, Lucerne, Switzerland
- Schilling Julian, Prof. MD, santésuisse, „Beauftragter für Qualitäts-Sicherung", Solothurn, Switzerland
- Tobler Jürg, Ex-Editor of newspaper „St.Galler Tagblatt", Meggen, Switzerland
- Trutmann Markus, MD, Editor Swiss Medical Publishers, Basel, Switzerland

Selected Reading

Bonnici AV, Koka SR, Richards DJ: Results of Buck screw fusion in grade 1 spondylolisthesis. JR Soc Med 1991;84:270–273.

Dutoit M, De Roguin B, Livio J: L4/5 spondylolisthesis following reduction and stabilization by anterior and posterolateral graft of L5/S1 spondylolisthesis with major displacement. Chir Pediatr 1987;28:256–258.

Frennered AK, Denielson BI, Nachemson AL, Nordwall AB: Midterm follow-up of young patients fused in situ for spondylolisthesis. Spine 1991;16:409–416.

Hacley JH: Degenerative lumbar spondylolisthesis with spinal stenosis: a prospective study comparing decompression with decopmpression and intertransverse process arthrodesis (letter). J Bone Joint Surg 1992;74B:426–430.

Hanley EN Jr: Decompression and distraction-deotation arthrodesis for degenerative spondylolisthesis. Spine 1986;11:269–276.

Jones AA, McAfee PC, Robinson RA, Zinreich SJ, Wang H: Failed arthrodesis of the spine for severe spondylolisthesis: salvage by interbody arthrodesis. J Bone Joint Surg (Am) 1988;70:25–30.

Kim NM, Kim DJ: Anterior interbody fusion for spondylolisthesis. Orthopedics 1991;14:1069–1076.

Knox BD, Harvell JC, Jr, Nelson BP, Hanley EN, Jr: Decompression and luyue rectangle fusion for degenerative spondylolisthesis. J Spinal Disord 1989;2:223–228.

Lack W, Eyb R, Leber H: The lateral profile of the lumbar vertebrae following lumosacral spondylodesis-comparision between Harrington rods and transpedicular fixation system (Zielke's method). Z Orthop 1989;129:19–24.

Lorenzz R: Lumbar spondylolistheis: clinical syndrome and operative experience with Cloward's technique. Acta Neurochir 1982;60:223–244.

Matzen KA: Ventral interligamental-intercorporal spondylodesis in spondylolisthesis. Z Orthop 1989;127:39–46.

Oh S, Sgier F: Knochenzapfen-Spondylodese bei lumbalem Wirbelgleiten. Z Inform Arzt 1999;409–416:12–13.

Oh S, Kim JB, Suh JK: Oblique posterior interbody fusion with bone plugs by unilateral apoproach for treamtne tof lumbar instability: technical notes. J Korean Neurosurg Soc 2003;33:525–527.

Stender W, Meissner HJ, Thomas W: Ventral interbody spondylodesis using a new plug-shaped implant. Neurosurg Rev 1990;13:25–34.

Takahashi K. Long-term results of anterior interbody fusion of treatment of degenerative spondylolisthesis. Spine 1990;15:1211–1215.

Valat JP, Eveleigh MC, Perrot Y, Fouquet B, Burdin P, Castaing J: Posterolateral arthrodiesis in spondylolisthesis and lumborsacral disk arthroses. Study of 11 cases with follow-up exceeding 5 years. Rev Rhum Mal Osteoartic 1987;54:567–573.

Subject Index